THE

THRIVING
CHILD

THE
THRIVING
CHILD

PARENTING SUCCESSFULLY THROUGH ALLERGIES, ASTHMA, AND OTHER COMMON CHALLENGES

ERICA REID

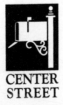

CENTER STREET

New York   Boston   Nashville

Center Street
Hachette Book Group
237 Park Avenue
New York, NY 10017

www.CenterStreet.com

Printed in the United States of America

RRD-C

First trade edition: August 2013
10 9 8 7 6 5 4 3 2 1

Center Street is a division of Hachette Book Group, Inc.
The Center Street name and logo are trademarks of Hachette Book Group, Inc.

The Hachette Speakers Bureau provides a wide range of authors for speaking events. To find out more, go to www.HachetteSpeakersBureau.com or call (866) 376-6591.

The publisher is not responsible for websites (or their content) that are not owned by the publisher.

The Library of Congress has cataloged the hardcover edition as follows:
Reid, Erica.
    The thriving child : parenting successfully through allergies, asthma, and other common challenges / Erica Reid.
        p. cm.
    ISBN 978-0-89296-864-0
    1. Children—Health and hygiene—Popular works.   2. Child rearing.   I. Title.
    RJ61.R414 2012
    649.1—dc23

                                                                              2011034048
ISBN 978-0-89296-863-3 (pbk.)

*This book of love and passion is dedicated to my Grandaddy,
my Nana, and all the children of the world, especially the ones
who made this possible,
Arianna Manuelle and Addison Kennedy Reid.
I love you all.*

Contents

Part II: An Emotionally Thriving Child

Dear Reader,

The Thriving Child is a labor of love. When you read this book, you and your child will benefit from the combined knowledge and experience of the many experts, on everything from pediatric immunology to child creativity, whom Erica Reid has assembled as her contributors. You'll also be treated to a wealth of information that Erica herself has uncovered, through years of painstaking research. And you'll find pages and pages of the kind of practical, real-world parenting tips that you can only get from a hands-on mom, who knows what it's like to try to convince a kid to eat a gluten-free cupcake while all the other kids have Twinkies.

Most of all, however, as you flip through the pages of *The Thriving Child*, you'll see an inspiring demonstration of a mother's love. As a practicing physician, I have met many parents who have confronted health challenges similar to those that Erica has faced, in raising a child with asthma and potentially severe food allergies. I know of no mother who has approached these challenges with a higher level of dedication than Erica. In these pages, you'll see that dedication reflected in Erica's exhaustive lists of food ingredients that you might not think to avoid, or of non-allergenic snacks that will keep long enough to take on an airplane trip. But you'll also see something of her heart and soul in this book, and of her unflagging commitment not just to keeping her kids medically well, but to nurturing them as whole human beings, and giving them every possible opportunity for physical, mental, and spiritual development.

In my medical training, I've come across much of the information about allergies, asthma, and nutrition that you'll find in this book, although there's plenty to learn here even for the professional. But it has only been through my own experience as a mother that I have truly come to appreciate the incredible rewards of parenthood, and the depth of devotion that can be expressed by committed parents. This book will help you to keep your kids healthy and out of the emergency room, but it will also do something perhaps even more important than that. It will help you teach them to live, learn, prosper and grow. In short, it will inspire you to help them thrive.

Sincerely,
Holly L. Phillips, MD

Foreword by Jennifer Lopez

I have been so blessed to have had my share of success in the worlds of music, movies, fashion design, TV, and more. But there is no question in my mind that the role I am most proud of, is being mother to my twins, Max and Emme. Mothering is one of the hardest jobs any woman can have.

I have always respected and looked up to mothers, especially my own. But it wasn't until I personally entered the unique world of motherhood that I began paying more attention to other mothers around me and seeking their insight. One of these women has been Erica Reid.

Erica and I met through her husband LA and our relationship has grown much closer with time. Not only are we two women who are friends, but two mothers. We spend a lot of time together with our children, enjoying meals, weekends, and family time. We help each other navigate through the unpredictable world of raising "coconuts." Having the objective eye of another mother can sometimes be the light you need to see clearly in the moments of uncertainty that arise on this motherhood journey. This has proven priceless to me. I can truly say that Erica is one of the most inspiring mothers I know.

As a working single mother of twins, it's an understatement to say that my plate is full. But despite a busy life, I try my best to make sure that my children receive what they need to sustain them both in their daily lives and in the long term. Life is truly what we make it and I feel that we all need a little help, especially when it comes to our children. As Erica mentions in this book, if your children aren't healthy and thriving, it doesn't matter how many awards you receive or how high profile your life is. This is why I find *The Thriving Child* to be such an important book. It is encouraging without being preachy, inspiring without being overwhelming, and it provides so much information that we as parents need in today's busy, fast-paced, high-tech world.

The Thriving Child gives practical tips from the actual experiences of a natural born mother. And the information isn't just helpful; I have seen it in action. I know that Erica walks the walk and talks the talk. I've even seen my own family benefit after time spent with her. (I know traveling with my kids has gotten easier thanks to a few of her key tips!) I'm excited that Erica has been generous enough to put pen to paper and share with others what she has experienced. I know her journey was not always easy. Almost losing her son to a deadly virus was one of the most painful moments of her life, one that still brings her to tears when she talks about it. And yet, she turned it into something positive and used it to help others. I know it will help you and your family. I truly feel that *The Thriving Child* will enhance the life of any mom looking for a little extra support now and then. And, after all, who doesn't need that. I know I do.

Lots of love,
Jennifer

Introduction

They say there's nothing like a mother's love. I came to truly understand that saying when one of my two children, who had just turned three, was fighting for his life battling a deadly strain of bacteria. When it happened, I realized the lengths we will go to in order to care for our children both physically and emotionally. Feeling like I was losing my son was my wake-up call. Before that, I had felt in control when it came to my kids. After all, up until they were toddlers I had been the one in charge of what they were eating and wearing, what time they went to bed, and whom they had playdates with. I made sure they washed their hands and took their baths. Nothing bad was going to happen to them because I was on top of it all. Or so I thought! For example, I nursed both my children, Arianna and Addison, for what I considered to be a substantial amount of time—twelve months and thirteen months, respectively. Because I had heard about all the research showing the health benefits of nursing, I thought they were never going to get sick—well, at least not at a young age.

Unfortunately, that was not the case. Yes, we did avoid the common cold, but not the ear infection or other, more serious things, as I will share with you in this book. The truly unexpected *can* happen. It happened to us. It was my wake-up call, an experience that taught me I am not as in control as I thought I was. It also taught me that putting my passion and energy into what I *can* control will help me raise children who are strong and healthy, both physically and emotionally. It will also help me become more aware as a mother and a human being.

It was my intuition that saved my son, Addison, when he was sick. (You'll hear more about that experience in chapter 2.) That inner voice now guides me in other areas of mothering beyond health, such as in disciplining my children and nurturing their self-esteem. I believe that mothers and fathers have to listen, really listen, to that voice, that insight and innate knowledge we all possess, to follow what we intuitively feel in our hearts. I want mothers and fathers everywhere to learn, as I did, to trust their intuition and stand up for their children. This will help them live healthier, richer, more productive lives—because no matter where you live, what you have, or what you do, no matter your race, class, religion, or beliefs, we all have one thing in common: we desire the best for our children.

In the following pages, I will share the unexpected journey I went on after Addison's illness, and the years of work it took to get where I am today. During that journey I read, I listened, I experimented—and I saw results. (And the journey is not over. Even today, I continue to research and gather information.) As the journey progressed, my passion became deeper and deeper. Will what I learned and what I've done work for everyone? No. And not all of it worked for my own children. But what I do know from having lived it is you can't find out what works until you try. I gained so much insight from my son's horrible emergency situation. But why wait until you have a life-threatening emergency to change your own life?

I'm not saying it was easy or quick, either—it wasn't—but in time it was rewarding, because many of the small steps I took reaped beneficial results, whether it was changing my children's diets, making my home a little greener, or being vocal at their schools. The changes in both my kids, and in me, were huge.

Mothers I knew—and even those I barely knew—who had seen or heard about the changes in my children came up to me at my kids' school and asked for advice about their own children. Others phoned or e-mailed me. It is so fulfilling to help, to have women I barely know call me to say thank you or to tell me excitedly about the changes they saw in their own children after doing just one small thing we'd discussed. Though each person had different concerns, most of them wound up saying, "You should write a book." I laughed this off, thinking, "Yeah, right. Me, of all people, write a book?"

But then my grandfather got sick. I went to visit him in the hospital, not knowing it would be the last time we saw each other. While I was sitting by his bedside he said, "Erica, I'm so proud of you. You have so much in you to give. I know you do." He died just a few days later. Something about his death turned a switch on inside of me. His words sparked a desire in me to share the information I had—information I had spent so much time and energy gathering. I realized that there were many kids in the world who could benefit from all I'd learned. I couldn't have all this information and selfishly keep it only for my two children when so many other kids could be helped, too. So I pulled out my computer and started writing. Mind you, I had no clue what I was doing, but that last conversation with my grandfather had gone somewhere deep within me. Maybe it was me grieving. Maybe it was a form of release. Maybe it was that someone as special as he was had had faith in me and had seen my passion. Or maybe I wanted to make him proud of me.

I didn't always know what that passion was. I'd always loved children, but that love became much more apparent once I had children of my own. Before I was a mom, I was a bit of a gypsy, traveling often, and always wondering what my purpose in life was. I was never serious about anything other than having fun, enjoying life, and seeing the world. It wasn't until I became a mother that I felt a sense of purpose in my life and realized that my passion was helping children—all children, not just my own. My kids taught me what real passion was just by being there for me to care for and nurture them.

I believe that the biggest reward we can receive as human beings is the blessing of a child, whether that child comes from the core of our bodies or from the love of our hearts. But we have to make sacrifices, and those sacrifices go beyond providing the basic necessities of food, shelter, and clothing. We have a role and a responsibility. We have to become aware and recognize the gift we've been given. Yes, it's a sacrifice, but it comes with the job. And the results can be amazing. Our outlook is the key.

I've always thought that things happen for a reason. Whether it is good or bad, I eventually figure out what that reason is. But when my son was sick, I seriously questioned this "things happen for a reason" theory. Today I think maybe the reason for that emergency situation was for me to share all this information with others.

As moms, as dads, as people, we all have so much power within us—each and every one of us. It wasn't given only to me. I'm not doing anything that the woman or man next door can't do. I'm the first person to say that I am no expert. I'm not a doctor. I don't have a degree in anything related to health. I do not know it all. And I certainly don't have all the answers. I've been trained only through firsthand experience and by the information I've gathered while raising children with allergies. I guess you could say I'm an expert in my own life and in what I've done for my own children—and that is the information I want to share.

Because I am not an expert or a doctor, I've included experts and doctors in this book. I've talked to highly respected professionals in various fields, many of whom helped me transform my life and the health of my children. You'll also hear from some celebrities, not because they are famous but because they are moms like us—wonderful, caring moms who, I think, have valuable insight to share. The truth is it doesn't matter if you have a TV show, Grammy-winning albums, or a number one movie at the box office, a mom is a mom. It doesn't matter how glitzy or glamorous your life is, when your children are sick or you have issues at their school, the red carpet and limo rides are yesterday's news.

The first half of this book talks about raising healthy children in a world full of allergens. Its primary focus is on health and nutrition. The second half of the book talks about how to create an emotionally thriving child, and by this I mean how to focus on the other areas that help a child thrive, such as teaching discipline, respect, and responsibilities; encouraging creativity in your kids; and teaching them to open their hearts. You don't have to focus on all these areas to reap results. Any changes you make will help, because taking one step is better than not taking any steps at all. This is a process, a work in progress, and it doesn't have to be difficult or radical. It is what you make it. Whatever advice or suggestions you take from this book, I hope they are as helpful to you as they have been to me and both my children. I've done some of your homework for you. Think of my children and me as your guinea pigs.

So get ready to change your life and your child's life for the better. Get excited. You can do it. I know you can. And I'm here to help.

Disclaimer: I cannot make promises. I am not guaranteeing that everything I write about, discuss, or advise in this book will give you the same experience or results I received for myself and my children. All I can do is share *my* experiences—the same things I've shared with friends, relatives, and other moms and dads at my kids' school—and explain what worked for us. I recommend that you use this book as a guide. I am no doctor of any sort. I am no expert of any sort. Nor am I perfect or trying to advise you as if I am. The experts I have selected to be part of this project are also speaking only from their own personal experiences and knowledge. I highly recommend that you seek professional help and answers from your go-to person, especially if you are dealing with certain health-related issues.

Whichever route you desire to take to care for yourself and your children, I wish you *only* great health—mentally, spiritually, and physically. Here's to your great health.

Thank you,

Erica Reid

PART I

A THRIVING CHILD IN A WORLD OF ALLERGENS

Chapter 1

Children Living with Food Allergies and Asthma

For any parent, I think you must first be well-informed before you speak to your child about his or her food allergies. I think the key, as it is in any other life lesson, is to be truthful, calm, and clear about the subject. Don't sugarcoat it, but at the same time teach your child that their food allergy is manageable, that they can successfully take the responsibility to be mindful and cautious, and that they don't have to live their life in fear. Knowledge is always power. There is no reason for a child with food allergies to feel left out or odd. They need to know what will hurt them and that they can live a full, normal life.

—Lori Stokes, mother of two

I will never forget the day my son was lying sick on the bathroom floor. Usually filled with boundless energy, twenty-two-month-old Addison was wrapped in a towel, his body limp and lethargic. His normally sparkling eyes, full of life, looked weak, and his typically glowing complexion was dull and pale. He was wiped out. I knew something was wrong. Really wrong. This wasn't a little cold or the latest bug going around. Addison's immune system was trying to fight something. *My child's sick. Really sick*, I thought as adrenaline raced through my body. Just moments earlier he'd been coughing, a deep, persistent cough that sounded like it was being caused by phlegm in his chest. I had turned on the shower and sat with him in the bathroom encouraging him to inhale the steam that surrounded us. I thought this would help break up the phlegm. But five minutes later, his cough was as deep as ever. Actually, it was worse, so I felt I'd made a mistake with the steam. I knew it was time to call our pediatrician.

"Bring him in," she said before I'd finished describing his symptoms.

I strapped Addison into his stroller and dashed the seven blocks to the doctor's office. (We live in New York City, where we walk and cab it everywhere.) I'd never moved down the street that fast in my life.

"He may have pneumonia," the pediatrician said after listening to Addison's chest. "Let's get a chest X-ray."

"An X-ray?" I asked.

"There's no other way to find out," she said. I hesitantly agreed. Then I strapped Addison in the stroller once again, left the pediatrician's office, and ran another seven blocks to the radiologist's office for the X-ray.

Before allowing Addison to sit on my lap, the X-ray technician diligently covered me with a heavy padded smock that went from my shoulders to the tops of my thighs. But nothing was used to protect my little boy. This made me feel uneasy. *If they're protecting me so carefully and I'm an adult, isn't all that radiation dangerous for his body?* I thought. But I had no choice and, like always, coached myself through it. *This is happening for a reason. I don't know why, but one day I will.* (Maybe it was to share my journey by writing this book.)

The X-ray confirmed my pediatrician's suspicion: Addison had pneumonia. "I'll call the drugstore with a prescription for an antibiotic," she said. I was amazed. My son wasn't even two years old and he was going from radiation exposure to getting his first antibiotic—a medication you're always told to use as infrequently as possible. Little did I know that this was the first of many antibiotics he'd be prescribed, and upper respiratory problems he'd have, and that I'd just taken my first step on an unexpected journey—because although

Addison did get better, the condition was never healed; the antibiotics were only a temporary fix, and the root cause of the problem was never addressed.

For the next year, Addison and I were in and out of different doctors' offices. He was having recurrent upper respiratory infections, and I was always told that it was bronchitis and that he had to have an antibiotic. This was not only frustrating, but upsetting and nerve-racking; I didn't like having to give him antibiotics so frequently and at such a young age. Aside from the fact that all these doctors' appointments were time-consuming, it was frustrating to have to share Addison's health history over and over again each time we saw a new doctor. One visit to a pulmonologist really stands out for me.

"He definitely has asthma," the doctor said after taking a family history. "Take this prescription and fill it immediately."

"What is it?" I asked.

"A nebulizer with a steroid," she said nonchalantly. It didn't feel as if her diagnosis and remedy were specifically for my child, but more robotic, automatic. She was doing exactly what she'd done with the patients who came in before my son, and would do the same with those who came after. Yes, I was prepared to hear that medication was the answer, but steroids? For a child who was under the age of two? I glanced over at my son, who was on the floor coloring. The thought of strapping a mask on his head and letting him inhale steroids into his tiny body was heartbreaking. Was this really the only way to help him? There was no other option here? This was a child who needed to build up his immune system, not fill it with chemicals.

"Come back in four weeks," the doctor said briskly, as if trying to wrap things up and move on to the next patient as fast as possible. *No way*, I thought. Something firm inside me was saying to her, *Your words are going in one ear and out the other. And nothing you suggest is going into my son's body!* I felt stubborn (more so than my usual stubborn self).

After this, a friend recommended that we see a well-known allergist at one of New York City's most prestigious hospitals. He was so busy that at that particular time there was a three-month wait to get an appointment with him. I was looking forward to meeting him, thinking this man with such a huge reputation would be able to help me find some answers.

When we finally got around to seeing him, he did some routine tests, including a skin test for some of the most common allergies such as peanuts, eggs, chocolate, and dairy. His conclusion? "For now, your son won't be able to do anything physical outside without two puffs of an albuterol inhaler every day," he said.

Albuterol is a medication that warns of asthma-related death on its label, so I wasn't particularly thrilled at this suggestion. I was also nervous because I recalled that the sister of supermodel Niki Taylor had lost her life after using an inhaler for her asthma. I didn't know the details of the story or if the inhaler was the official cause of death, but that tragic story stood out in my mind and raised a red flag for me.

Next, the doctor handed me a stack of prescriptions: one for the inhaler, one for a nebulizer, a third for steroids, and the last for an EpiPen, an injectable device that contains the drug epinephrine, which he said Addison couldn't leave home without.

"Why an EpiPen?" I asked.

"Your son is highly allergic to eggs."

"But he eats eggs and he's fine," I protested. Addison had never had an allergic reaction to eggs, and certainly not the hives, shortness of breath, or swollen lips that would have warranted the use of an EpiPen.

"He's highly allergic," the doctor repeated, an air of frustration in his voice. "His tests revealed that he's allergic to egg."

I continued trying to convince him otherwise, but he didn't seem to hear a word I was saying. Instead he dismissed me. I wasn't surprised. During the appointment he had been racing back and forth between my son and the patient in the room next door. He was on autopilot. Not once did he look me in the eye or show any compassion or patience. Though he said very little, his whole manner spoke loud and clear. It told me, *You're the patient. I'm the doctor. Just sit there, be quiet, and accept my help.* Not once did I feel that I was being heard or did he slow down long enough for me to say, "What do you mean?" And this was the famous doctor who had a three-month-long waiting list! Just like the immunologist we'd seen before, he was stuck in a routine and made me feel like Addison was just a number.

That appointment revved up my engine. From the moment I stepped out of that doctor's office, I was on a mission. *I can't and I will not just take someone else's word,* I thought. *There must be something else I can do to help my son deal with these health issues. What are the options? Keep him medicated? Shots? Something natural? Get a second opinion?* And that was the start of my trying to find alternative remedies for the medications these doctors wanted to prescribe for my child. A child who had yet to celebrate his second birthday!

Knowing there was something else out there for Addison besides steroids, but unclear what that "something" was, I started to do research. I went directly from that doctor's office to a health food store. After all, if I was being urged to take a chance with prescription medications, it couldn't hurt to take a chance first with something with no side effects. At the health food store, I perused the aisle of books, pulled one off the shelf, and put it on the counter.

"That book's okay," said the store owner. "But this one is great." He pointed to *The Allergy and Asthma Cure: A Complete 8-Step Nutritional Program* by Dr. Fred Pescatore. I was intrigued. It sounded like what I was looking for.

"Thank you," I said, grateful that someone was actually trying to help me. I was so taken aback by the title of Pescatore's book that to this day I don't remember the name of the first book I'd selected. All I remember is that I put it back on the shelf, grabbed Dr. Pescatore's book, paid for it, and headed home.

Later, my kids and I went through our usual nightly routine of dinner, baths, and bedtime stories. Though I usually savored our bedtime ritual, that night I was eager to curl up with my new book and hopefully find something—even just one piece of insightful information. And I did. I read the book from cover to cover, so absorbed, highlighting so much information, that the next thing I knew it was 1:00 a.m. I knew I needed to sleep, because soon enough I'd have to wake up and start the day with two young children. But I was too wide-eyed and excited. Everything this man was saying made sense. He was talking *to me*. He was talking about *my son*! I flipped the book over to see where the author was located and was amazed to find that he had an office right in New York City. I wanted to make sure he was still in practice, so I called information for his number and then called his office. (Yes, I knew no one was going to answer at one in the morning, but I wanted confirmation that this was the right place.) When I heard, "You've reached the office of Dr. Fred Pescatore," I was elated. The next morning, the first thing I did was call again and make an appointment. I brought Addison in days later (and my daughter after that), and we've been seeing Dr. Pescatore ever since. I can honestly say that this man has helped change our lives.

At that first appointment, Dr. Pescatore did a blood test for food allergies. (The last doctor had done only skin tests, which aren't believed to be as accurate.) Even before that appointment with Pescatore, I knew Addison was allergic to milk and soy, something I'd discovered when he was an infant. I had nursed both of my children, but Addison ate a lot, so I never had enough breast milk to pump and store in the freezer for him. This was a problem if I had to go out and someone else had to feed him. I had needed a backup plan. Our pediatrician had suggested a milk-based formula, but my son broke out with a little reddish-colored rash on his cheeks immediately after I gave it to him. Obviously, he was reacting to something. When I gave him soy milk, the same thing happened.

Dr. Pescatore's more thorough testing revealed that Addison was allergic to more than a dozen foods! The list the doctor handed me, along with a color-coded chart, included black pepper, vanilla, cinnamon, and wheat. This was surprising at first. I'd never heard of anyone being allergic to some of those things (black pepper?). I was even more surprised when Dr. Pescatore told me to omit these foods completely from my son's diet. "Just try it for three months," he said.

He tried to reassure me, but honestly, I wanted to cry. All I was thinking was, *How is it really possible to avoid all those foods? I'm no chef.* I hesitated, because this was a lot to do. But once I set those feelings aside, I agreed, even though I really wasn't sure that I had it in me to do this. This task felt beyond overwhelming. But I thought about my son and his health instead of thinking about what I wanted to do.

At that point I did know a little bit about food allergies. All my life I'd been allergic (like my mother before me) to tree nuts (the only "nuts" I can eat are peanuts, which aren't technically nuts, but legumes), fish, and seafood. As a result, I grew up very aware that I had to be careful. My daughter is also allergic to nuts, which I discovered when she was a baby. Still, dealing with nut and fish allergies is very different from dealing with a son with a long list of foods—common foods that are everywhere—to avoid.

I'll be honest. I've been doing this for five years now, and at times it is still overwhelming to have to monitor my children's food intake and be on guard for a reaction. At times it's challenging. But so are many other things in life—such as marriage and work—and I believe that it's all in how you choose to go in there and tackle it. If you're trying to move up the job ladder at work, you have to roll up your sleeves and put in some hard work. You have to educate yourself, to learn. I don't see this as any different. I had to make myself aware and knowledgeable. I can't focus on the fact that I have to study every food label or fill my purse with special food and medication every time we leave the house. Am I going to get upset and angry? No, because that won't take away my children's, or my, food allergies. They are a part of who we are, but they don't define us. I try to focus on the positive: my son may have a lot of allergies, but they are manageable. He doesn't have to live in a bubble, and it could be a lot worse.

Allergies are more prevalent today than ever before, so you *can* find foods made without eggs, gluten, or dairy, and many labels tell you if a product was made in a facility with nuts or other allergy-causing ingredients. Plus, more people are aware of food allergies today than ever before. For example, my son certainly has it better than I did when I was his age. When I was growing up, I was the only kid in class with food allergies. Today, I know so many people whose children have allergies and asthma. Some cases are mild; some are severe. In short, those of us with food allergies are not alone.

Researchers from the University of Pittsburgh discovered that allergic reactions caused by food led to more than 7 million emergency room visits during the period 2001–2005. That's an average of 203,000 each year! Ninety thousand of those were for the potentially life-threatening allergic reaction called anaphylaxis.

This is why I want to share whatever knowledge I've discovered on my journey, because I know that every little bit helps. What follows are the things that have made living with my children's allergies and my own safer and easier for all of us.

Take Your Time Introducing New Foods

When Arianna was six months old, her pediatrician, Dr. Barbara Landreth, told me she was ready to try eating solid foods. Dr. Landreth gave me a feeding chart and told me to give my daughter just one food for two to three days, because that's a good way to check for food allergies. This was long before I knew Arianna had any allergies and two years before Addison was born.

I'd heard other pediatricians suggest offering your child different foods all at once, but I liked Dr. Landreth's more conservative and careful approach. This was also the approach I took with Addison, because by the time he was starting to eat solid foods, I knew he was allergic to dairy and maybe sensitive to soy. So I took my time, introduced one food for two to three days, and watched for a reaction. The reasoning behind this is that if you give a child a few foods at a time and he has a reaction, you won't know which food was the problem. I strongly suggest you try this. It is very helpful.

Look for Subtle Signs

With allergies, we all look for the well-known reactions, the ones that are obvious, such as hives, swelling of the face, or the inability to breathe. But there are subtler signs of allergies or asthma. For example, my son ate eggs without a problem until he was around four to five years old. Then one day I gave him a fried egg. Instantly, he started snorting, and his nose was running—something that wasn't normal on an eighty-degree summer day. This, it turned out, was a subtle sign of an allergy. Other subtle signs of an allergy include sneezing, coughing, throat itching, a headache, a skin rash, and an eczema breakout, among others. After that, I took him off all foods with eggs in them. No cake, no cookies. At that point his diet was already wheat-free, dairy-free, and gluten-free. Now it was egg-free.

When Addison had that reaction to the fried egg, I thought back to the doctor who'd told me Addison was allergic to eggs, even though he seemed fine eating them. It turns out, as I have since learned, that you can become allergic to a food you've already been eating for a while. (More on this in the "Answers from Erica's Expert" section of this chapter.) Since then I have found out that Addison is allergic not to the entire egg but only to the white part. No doctor had told me that it is possible to be allergic to the yolk of the egg and not the egg white or vice versa. Normally when you think "egg," you don't think to separate the yolk from the white.

Read Food Labels

I read labels carefully and have tried to learn the alternate names for foods and ingredients that my kids and I are allergic to. For example, you can't have palm oil if you're allergic to certain seeds. And a food label that may not explicitly say the food has milk in it may in fact contain milk, as there are other words that mean milk, like dairy, or milk protein, like casein. I discovered this when I gave Addison rice cheese, thinking it was dairy-free, and he had a reaction. I researched the product further and learned that rice cheese contains a milk protein called casein.

If I have any doubts at all about a food, we don't eat it. I like to be on this side of caution. If I'm not clear about what an ingredient means, and I can't Google it or ask someone who knows, then I don't let my kids eat it. Period. It's just not worth the potentially fatal risk.

Talk to Your Children About Their Allergies

This is important for a few reasons: First, I don't want my children to feel that there's something wrong with them or that their allergies were caused by something they did. Nothing is wrong with them and they did not do anything to cause their problem. Their allergies are just part of them, not something they asked for. I talk to my kids about their allergies. I do not make a big deal about it, but I want to inform them. Second, they need to know about their allergies because that information just might save their lives. For example, my son knows not to eat or drink anything at a playdate, party, or at school, and he knows to ask if a food is okay for him if he's never eaten it before or if he is unaware or unsure he's had it before.

Don't Leave Home Without Supplies

I never want to be caught unprepared. We live in New York City, where many stores are open 24-7 and where there are drugstores every few blocks, but I still keep important medications and other items on me at all times. It's too risky to assume that I can race to the store in the event of an emergency, so I never leave home without the following:

- **An EpiPen.** I keep one in my purse, one in the car, and one in a kitchen cabinet. If my husband, kids, and I are attending an event and I am carrying a smaller purse (the kind that has just enough room to fit a cell phone, driver's license, lip gloss, and cash), I carry with me a few pre-measured, packaged spoons of Benadryl (they are called Children's Benadryl Allergy Perfect Measure pre-filled spoons) and an EpiPen. Get the dual EpiPen package, which contains two EpiPens and a practice EpiPen in one box. That way, if you mess up with one EpiPen, you'll have a backup. I also regularly check the expiration dates of any medications, such as our EpiPens and Benadryl. When they've expired, I make sure to replace them.

- **EpiPen instructions.** You and your child may know how to work your EpiPen—and if you don't, practice, maybe on an orange, before an emergency occurs—but in the case of an allergic attack, you may not be the ones using it. A friend, teacher, or babysitter may be the person on hand to use it on your child, so keeping the instructions with the EpiPen is critical. (Note: Once you've used an EpiPen on your child, take him to the emergency room right afterward, because of the effect the medication can have on the heart and to make sure your child has received enough of the medication. The dose from the EpiPen may not carry him through, so he'll need to be monitored to stop flare-ups. Though I carried an EpiPen for years, I didn't know this until I was an adult.)

- **Benadryl.** The use of medication is not my first choice, but if my kids' mouths are itching, it may be an allergic reaction. For this, I give them Benadryl. I'm not going to play around. For me, Benadryl is like a credit card: I never leave home without it. This wasn't always the case. It wasn't until I had children with allergies that I thought to carry an EpiPen and Benadryl at all times for my own allergies. I have a few purses I use regularly, so I buy a box of Benadryl and put at least three pills in each purse, so if I switch bags at the last minute, I'm still covered. (And who knows? Someone else may need one, too.) The company that makes Benadryl also makes liquid Benadryl, with pre-measured spoons that are individually wrapped, so you don't have to carry a big bottle with you. Because liquid is absorbed into the blood-stream faster than pills, this is my first choice, so I carry both pills and liquid.

- **Albuterol inhaler.** I rarely ever use this for my son, but you never know what's around the corner. Situations can arise, and I have to be smart, realistic, and prepared. I always take the inhaler on vacations, just in case (and have had to use it on Addison while traveling).

- **Medical bracelets.** My kids wear medical bracelets that list what they're allergic to and give my cell phone number. It's a precaution I take, because you can never know what will happen. For example, if I drop them at a kids' club on vacation, I may tell one caregiver there that the kids have allergies, but another caregiver may come in later and not be given this information. The bracelets are just another pre-caution, another way to make everyone aware. And nowadays they come in many cute styles, so kids don't mind wearing them.

- **Your own food.** I can't take a chance that a store, birthday party, air-port, or plane will have something that my kids can eat, so my purse is always stocked with acceptable snacks. When we're traveling, I bring more than I think we'll need, so I'm ready in case of a flight delay or unexpected traffic. (More on that in chapter 7.) I carry these snacks in my purse because I live in New York City and don't drive a car. But if you're in your car a lot, keep it stocked with snacks. When we travel by plane, I always bring extra food, and this often includes applesauce and soy yogurt. Because these foods have a bit of a liquid consistency, they're not normally allowed through airport security. So I carry a signed and dated letter from Addison's doctor explaining Addison's life-threatening food allergies and that he needs to carry food with him on the plane. This has been a huge help on several occasions.

Make Living with Allergies/Asthma Easier for Your Kids

AT HOME

Obviously having so many food allergies makes it difficult for my children to eat in certain circumstances. As a result, I make sure that our home is the one place that's safe for us all. My daughter wants to have what she calls "real food," such as ice cream or regular (not spelt) bagels, but in my opinion our home needs to be the one safe haven for all of us to eat freely and comfortably. As a result, I purchase only what we can *all* eat and not all that we want to eat. I want to be able to leave my house and not worry that someone who doesn't know any better is pouring cow's milk for Addison rather than rice milk or giving him the wrong cheese. The minute Addison leaves our home, we have to be concerned, so I don't want him to have to feel that when he is in the comfort of his own home. Yes, it's a sacrifice that we don't have nuts, cow's milk, or cheese in our kitchen, and it may not be what others in my home want, but we have to set those feelings aside so our home is safe for all of us.

IN THE SCHOOL CAFETERIA

My son's school offers only one option for lunch: their cafeteria food. You can't bring your own lunch from home. School rule. (Crazy, I know, especially in today's world of food allergies.) But because the school can't accommodate Addison's food allergies with the foods they offer, he is allowed to bring his own lunch to school, but only with a doctor's note saying he has to do so. I don't want him to feel singled out or different, so each month I get the school's lunch menu and each morning I pack him a healthier version of what the rest of the kids will be eating that day. For example, if the meal for the day is turkey tacos and oatmeal-raisin cookies, I make him a turkey taco with organic turkey meat and organic corn taco shells and bake him oatmeal-raisin cookies that contain no dairy, no eggs, no nuts, no gluten, no wheat, and no sugar. (They're simply sweetened with agave or maple syrup and lots of mother's love. See the recipe on page 229.) If the school is serving pizza, I defrost a frozen gluten-free, dairy-free pizza the night before and bake it the next morning. If they're having ravioli, I pack ravioli made with tofu, which I get at the health food store. No, I don't always match the school's lunch exactly, and yes, this is time-consuming. It's also not the easiest thing to do when I'm rushing to get two kids up and out the door. But it's better than letting my son starve or feel ostracized.

I also make sure that his teacher has a stash of sweets that he can eat so if someone unexpectedly brings in a treat for the class, the teacher can pull out his treats and he won't feel left out. If I know in advance that it's a classmate's birthday and that child is bringing in cupcakes, I pack a gluten-free, dairy-free, egg-free cupcake for Addison, which I bake or purchase from a specific bakery here in New York City that makes treats he can eat.

AT PARTIES

If my son goes to a birthday party, he brings his own food. Before the party, I call the parents to find out what they're serving for the main meal—which is usually chicken nuggets and pizza. (See "Alternative Birthday Party Menu" on page 238.) I also ask if they're having cake or cupcakes for dessert. Armed with this information, I then provide versions of these foods that Addison can eat. There are times when I forget to call the parents or don't have time to make his food. In that case, he knows not to eat anything served at the party, and I give him one of the snacks that is always stashed in my purse.

WHILE TRAVELING

When we travel, I often try to find a local health food store and buy food that Addison can eat, such as rice milk, frozen waffles, and his favorite ice-cream sandwiches. Then I'll ask the hotel kitchen to keep these items and deliver them when we order room service. This way when we order breakfast or dessert, Addison can feel included in the room service delivery and I can be certain that what he's eating is safe for him.

Inform Everyone of Your Child's Allergies

AT SCHOOL OR ON A PLAYDATE

Wherever my kids go, be it school or a playdate, I call the adult who will be watching them to let her know which foods each of my children is allergic to. Because of Addison's extensive list of allergies, I tell that parent not to give him anything—no food, no drinks, no gum or candy. Not even water. I want that parent to know how serious the situation is. Unless a caregiver has a child with that specific allergy, or is allergic to that food herself, I can't assume she'll know this. I also can't assume she will be able to figure out what foods not to give my child. So I make it easier for her and for Addison by simply saying, "Don't give him anything." Then I pack him a snack and a drink.

I also make sure that anyone who supervises my children knows how to use an EpiPen. I can't just assume they'll be able to figure it out.

IN A RESTAURANT OR AT A PARTY

When we're at a restaurant, dinner party, or anywhere I'm not preparing the food for myself or my children, I always make a point of notifying the people preparing and serving our food that we have severe food allergies, and I inquire if the things we are allergic to are included in the items they're serving. At restaurants, I make sure that the person taking our order fully understands that we have serious, life-threatening allergies. When I order, I even ask the waiter to repeat the order, because I can never be sure what he's actually writing down. For example, once on a trip to Florida I made sure the woman answering our call for hotel room service wrote down that our meals had to be made without nuts, fish, cream, dairy, or butter. I also had her write down that we were allergic to these foods. If she hadn't, it might have looked as if we're just being picky and those preparing the food might not have been as careful in eliminating those ingredients from our meals.

If a waiter, party hostess, or event planner isn't completely certain about the ingredients in our meal, I have them ask the person preparing the food. (You can even carry cards with you that say what kind of allergy you have and ask your waiter to give one to the person preparing your food. You can make your own laminated card from index cards. And be sure to put your photo on them so they know which person at the table has the food allergy. Or you can get allergy cards off the Internet that list what you're allergic to. You can add your photo to these, too.)

Sometimes I even inform the manager or maître d' of a restaurant of our food allergies. You have to stay on top of this to help prevent mistakes.

I also take note of everything on the plate when the food is served, because an allergen may not be in our food, but could be used as a garnish. This happened to us on a vacation when we ordered room service. Our dessert came with what looked like brown sugar sprinkled around the edge of the plate. Even though the waiter assured us it was brown sugar, my gut told me to ask someone else. And I'm glad I did, because after a lot of back-and-forth with the kitchen, we learned that the garnish was in fact nuts. What saved us was my listening to my intuition.

I've also learned to make sure that anyone bringing food to our table in a restaurant knows about our allergies. For example, I may tell the waiter about our situation, but that doesn't mean the person who brings the bread basket to the table is aware of it. This happened to me when we were on vacation. I told the waiter I was allergic to nuts, but not the person who brought the bread basket. So there I was enjoying a nice piece of bread when I realized, too late, that it had nuts in it. I immediately had a reaction, which included an itchy mouth, itchy lips, and a racing heart (because I was so nervous). In the end, we had to rush out of the restaurant without anyone finishing their meal and call around to find a local doctor who would make a house call. It may sound like a lot of effort to have to inform the employees of a restaurant about your child's allergies, but it can be a matter of life and death.

IN A FOREIGN COUNTRY

If you're traveling to a place where you don't speak the language, it's a good idea to learn how to say your allergies in that particular language. Or have someone write the words for your allergies down on a piece of paper in that language so that you can show this to waiters, chefs, and anyone else handling your food.

Educate Your Child's School

Each school has a different policy when it comes to food allergies, so you have to research what foods your child's school does and does not allow to enter the school building, and how strict they are about enforcing this. If your school is lax about enforcing an anti-allergen policy—and even if they are not—here are some things you should do to protect your child:

- On the first day of school, communicate to the teachers about your child's allergies. So what if they look at you like you are a crazy, over-reactive parent. Food allergies are serious, and if you don't treat them that way, the school won't either. After all, it's your duty to speak up for your child.
- Make sure the school nurse and your child's teachers know what to do in case of an allergy attack, such as how to use an EpiPen or how much Benadryl to dispense. Don't assume they know about allergies or asthma, because unless they or loved ones have allergies, they may not know what to do.
- Have your child's teacher tell other parents in the class about your child's allergies, so that they can try not to bring foods with those ingredients for in-class birthdays or celebrations.
- Find out whom your child sits next to at lunch. For example, if that child tends to bring peanut butter and jelly for lunch and your child is allergic to peanuts, you may have to get that seat reassigned. This is especially important if your child customarily has a reaction to a food even if that food is simply in the same room or if their skin comes in contact with it.

There is a link between being bullied and having food allergies. A recent study in the *Annals of Allergy, Asthma and Immunology* found that an estimated 24 percent of kids who have food allergies have been bullied, teased, or harassed as a result.* They're teased about what they eat or about what they can't eat. And the teasing is not only verbal; it can be physical, with the bully sometimes throwing or waving the allergenic food, or touching the allergic child with it. Make this information known to your school's principal and other officials.

Listen to Your Intuition

I have learned to do this *most* of the time, but I have my moments when I do not listen hard enough. This happened on a recent vacation. We were at the beach, and Addison ran into a friend he had met the previous year. After they had played together for a while, the boy's mother told me they were going into town to get ice cream and she asked if Addison could join them. I said okay, but told her that he was allergic to dairy, so he could have only sorbet, *not* ice cream. Then I told Addison that our babysitter needed to go with him. This wasn't because I didn't trust the parents or needed the babysitter to watch Addison play with his friend. It was because our babysitter knows what he's allergic to, what to watch for, and what to do in case of a reaction. I also wanted her there because I knew that if he did have a reaction, he would be more comfortable going to her than to his friend's mom, whom he barely knew.

But once I said that the babysitter had to go along, Addison got really frustrated. "Why does someone always have to go with me on a playdate?" he protested. "How come I can't go with a friend and no adult from our family?"

I understood his frustration, and it was hard to see him so upset. But, as always, I explained to him that I wasn't going to send him out for ice cream without an adult who was familiar with his food allergies. I explained that his friend's parents didn't have a child with food allergies (I had asked) and that I didn't want to give them the responsibility, in the event of an allergy attack,

---

* *Annals of Allergy, Asthma and Immunology*, Volume 104, Edition 4: "Bullying Among Pediatric Patients with Food Allergy" by Jay A. Lieberman, Christopher Weiss, Terence J. Furlong, Mati Sicherer, Scott H. Sicherer; pp. 282–286.

to know what to look for and what to do. "People from our home know, but that's not the case for many people," I told him.

Addison and I argued back and forth. I was so torn. He was so frustrated. I felt for him. I knew he just wanted time with his friend without a babysitter. He persisted and persisted. Finally, I agreed. But first I looked him straight in the eye, pointed my index finger directly at him, and said firmly, "You can go this time, and this time only. But do not ask again. This is the one time and this is it." He was thrilled. I was nervous. I reiterated to the parents that he could have *only sorbet*. Then I sent them on their way with our Benadryl and my child.

One reason I let Addison go was that my husband and I were heading to the same place anyway, even though Addison and his friend's family were going to arrive before us. But shortly after they left, I got a strange feeling. Something wasn't right. I was already uncomfortable with the decision I had made, and now I had this strong sense that my son needed me. At this point, we were stuck in slow-moving traffic. The slower the cars moved, the faster my heart beat. Finally, I turned to my husband and said, "I'm getting out of the car and walking." Actually, I started running (we were in a small Caribbean town, so it's not as if I were running on a freeway or for blocks). When I walked into the ice-cream place, it took a second for me to find Addison. Then I saw him: sitting at a table with his friend and the friend's parents. He was spitting into a napkin. When he saw me, he jumped up and walked up to meet me. "Mommy, my tongue is itching," he said. "My tongue is itching." I ran over to the table and looked at the cup he had been eating from. One look at the creamy texture and I could immediately tell it wasn't sorbet; it was ice cream.

I dumped my whole purse onto the nearest table, not caring that everything from pens to tampons came spilling out. I was looking for the Benadryl and hoping this moment would require only Benadryl, not an EpiPen or a visit to the emergency room at an unfamiliar local hospital on a little Caribbean island. When I found the Benadryl, I gave it to Addison, and then took him to the bathroom. As I stood there washing out his mouth and wiping his lips, I was crying, saying to him (and to myself), "I knew better. I knew better. I knew not to let you go alone. This is why I wanted the babysitter to go with you."

His friend's parents apologized profusely, but I knew it wasn't their fault. It was mine. We'd been going to that place since Addison was a baby, and nothing like this had ever happened. But I had let my guard down. I hadn't listened to that little voice inside me saying, *Send the babysitter.* It was a difficult moment, but I believe every situation offers a lesson. That day the lesson was to continue to follow my instincts whenever that inner voice spoke to me. Addison learned a lesson, too. We learned it the hard way, at the same time and together.

Even with a food allergy, your children *can* eat their favorite foods. You just have to learn how to make them without the ingredients that cause a reaction in them. For example, I've had to learn to make dairy-free, egg-free, sugar-free cookies, because I do not want my son to feel deprived and I want him to eat better-quality food. (I know these treats don't sound very delicious, but they are. See the recipes in "Really Easy Recipes Your Kids Will Love.") After all these years of having children with allergies, and dealing with my own, I now try to take a recipe and tweak it so it works for us. It takes a few tries to get it right, but when it's right, oh my gosh, it's so yummy. I'm not someone who enjoys cooking, but I enjoy knowing that my kids are eating healthy foods that they can benefit from. As a result, I have surprised them and myself with some of my edible discoveries.

ANSWERS FROM ERICA'S EXPERT

Fred Pescatore, MD, is a traditionally trained physician who practices nutritional medicine and is the author of several well-known books on the subject, such as *The Allergy and Asthma Cure, Feed Your Kids Well, Boost Your Health with Bacteria*, and the *New York Times* bestseller *The Hamptons Diet*. Pescatore is president of the International and American Associations of Clinical Nutritionists and the head of Medicine 369, an integrative medical facility in New York City.

Allergies

What is an allergy?

Allergies are now the most common chronic disease in North America and are more prevalent than heart disease or diabetes. A broad definition is an abnormal, adverse physical reaction of the body to certain substances known as allergens. Allergy sufferers usually react to quantities of allergens that leave most people unharmed. Some allergies are defined by what causes them, such as a food allergy or insect allergy, while others are defined by their symptoms, such as hay fever, hives, or eczema.

What are the most common food allergies?

Ninety percent of all food allergies are to milk; peanuts; soy; eggs; nuts, such as cashews, almonds, or walnuts (peanuts are actually legumes); shellfish; fish; or wheat. Peanuts, fish, shellfish, and nuts usually cause the most severe reactions.

What's the difference between a skin prick test and a blood test for allergies?

Skin prick testing is what most people are familiar with and remains the primary diagnostic procedure to determine the cause of allergies in this country. Here, an allergen is injected into the surface of the skin, usually on the back of the forearm, upper arm, or upper back. The allergen interacts with specific antibodies on the surface of your skin mast cells. If you're allergic to the substance, this will trigger the release of histamines and redness and/or swelling about fifteen minutes after you were injected. Skin prick tests are limited because they measure only an immediate hypersensitivity to antibodies called IgE. If this isn't the kind of allergy you have, the test will be negative, but you still may be allergic to the allergen tested. The results of this test are also dependent on the person performing it. Factors such as the amount of allergen used; the depth, angle, and force of the needle; and the stability of the allergen extracts can cloud results.

Blood tests attempt to isolate your food sensitivities and allergies using your blood. There are several different types of blood tests. In the one I use most frequently, your blood is incubated with the individual allergens in separate little containers—each for a different food. The reactions that this test measures are multifaceted. Different components of the immune system that may all lead to inflammation, and hence to allergies and asthma, are measured. This is the main reason I think this test is important.

What's the difference between a food allergy and food sensitivity?

A food sensitivity is only going to make you uncomfortable and cause symptoms you may not even realize are related to the food, such as a headache, runny nose, stomachache, brain fog, and, for kids, not being able to sit still. The tricky part is that it can take up to seventy-two hours before you actually experience these symptoms, so oftentimes you can't identify the culprit. Also, there are around three hundred symptoms that can be related to food sensitivities. They are not life threatening, but they can be troublesome and, in my opinion, are an underlying cause of asthma, allergic rhinitis (hay fever), eczema, hives, and even acne.

A food allergy is much more dramatic. If you have a food allergy, the reaction to that food will be very immediate, and can also be quite deadly. For example, your throat will close up, you can get hives, or your lips can swell. Other reactions include sneezing and coughing.

If you find out that you have a food sensitivity, do you have to give that food up forever?

No. You should avoid the foods for which you test positive for three to six months. You don't have to eliminate those foods forever—just until your body has had time to heal and for the inflammation to be reduced. Three to six months may seem like a long time, but the inflammatory process in your body took a long time to develop and needs some time to heal. Be patient.

How does someone develop an allergy to something that just years before they weren't allergic to?

Allergies can strike at any time, usually without warning. You may go your whole life without any allergies and then develop them. The way it happens is very complicated, but basically your body can build up antibodies to certain foods—usually the ones you eat most often—so your body will become sensitized to those foods. Therefore, the minute you eat those things again, your body immediately recognizes them as foreign, and an inflammatory reaction takes place more quickly.

Asthma

What is asthma?

An estimated 4.8 million children in the United States have asthma, the number one chronic respiratory disease in North America. It's a disease of the lungs, in which the tubes inside the lungs that deliver air, known as bronchi, become inflamed. When this happens, the muscles of the bronchial walls tighten and extra mucus is produced, causing the airway to narrow. Asthma attacks can range in severity from slight wheezing to life threatening. Fifty to 80 percent of children with asthma will have symptoms before the age of five.

Why are allergies and asthma in kids more prevalent today than they used to be?

I think the reason is twofold. One big theory that has been proven many, many times in European studies is that we're too clean. We clean, sterilize, and disinfect everything these days—especially around young children. As a result, the immune system doesn't get an opportunity to work when you're young, a time when the body is developing its immune defense strategy. So if it doesn't have anything to develop against, you're going to be more prone to things such as allergies and asthma.

Number two is the fact that our food supply is so severely damaged. We're not nourishing our bodies. We're actually de-nourishing them with all the processed foods and with crops such as wheat, soy, and corn that are genetically modified today. For example, wheat today doesn't resemble the wheat our ancestors ate just one hundred years ago. Because of this, we're chronically stressing the body, leaving it open to inflammatory conditions such as allergies and asthma. Unfortunately, it's difficult to get around this, because often food that's not genetically modified or healthier is more expensive or not available in some areas.

What's the link between allergy and asthma?

Allergies can often cause asthma attacks and make asthma worse. But not everyone with allergies will have asthma. The reason they are often talked about together is that they're both highly inflammatory conditions. They're the body's expression of the internal inflammation that's going on.

What are the differences between allergies and asthma?

Though the symptoms tend to overlap, here are some important differentiations.

ALLERGY:

- Is characterized by fatigue, headache, runny nose, stuffy nose, sneezing, postnasal drip, itchy and watery eyes, scratchy throat
- May occur only during specific seasons or year-round
- Is a specific trigger for the symptoms
- Is successfully treated with medications

ASTHMA:

- Is characterized primarily by shortness of breath, wheezing, and coughing
- Is not a single condition but may be mild, moderate, or severe, and can be intermittent or persistent
- Can be allergic, nonallergic, exercise induced, drug induced, cold air induced, or occupational

What are the signs to look for to know if your child has asthma?

The most common signs include coughing, wheezing, difficulty breathing, labored breathing, shortness of breath, constricted chest, panting, or these symptoms being triggered by something specific, such as allergens, cold air, or playing sports.

If my child doesn't have any of these signs, could he still have asthma?

Yes. There are certain warning signs that often precede a full-blown asthma attack by a few hours. They are unusual fatigue, a tight feeling in the chest, dry mouth, mouth breathing, sudden coughing, rapid heartbeat, anxiety, irritability, scratchy throat, and perspiration.

Do asthma symptoms vary from person to person?

Absolutely. Most of them will be very common, yet I have found them to be quite variable among my patient population.

What are some common asthma and allergy triggers?

Aerosol sprays, air pollution, animal dander, certain medications (such as aspirin or ibuprofen), cockroaches, cold outdoor temperatures, dust mites, estrogen, exercise, foods, gastroesophageal reflux disease or heart-burn, heredity, molds (indoor and outdoor), obesity, perfumes and other chemicals, pollens, respiratory and sinus infections, smoke, strong emotions, sulfites (preservatives in red wine, beer, dehydrated soups, some items in salad bars, and other foods), thunderstorms, and viruses.

What's the difference between mild, moderate, and severe asthma?

People with asthma can be split up into mild, moderate, and severe cases, depending on their symptoms. Those with mild asthma comprise 50 percent of the asthmatic population. They have symptoms only once or twice per year and are generally controlled on "as needed" bronchodilator medications. Forty percent of all patients with asthma fall into the moderate category. These people have symptoms roughly once per month, and some require daily medication to keep their symptoms from getting worse and interfering with their daily lives.

Severe asthma is a life-threatening form of this condition. The severe types usually require multiple daily medications just to maintain decent control over their breathing. Wheezing and coughing occur most of the time, and these patients usually find it difficult to participate in sporting activities.

Is asthma preventable?

That's a good question. If there's a family history of asthma and allergies, then I think it can be preventable if you take steps very early in your child's life to make sure she is tested for allergies, including food sensitivities. It's also pre-ventable if we don't keep our kids in a world where we clean, sterilize, and disinfect everything. We need to let them get dirty and be exposed to germs, because it's the only way their immune systems learn to work.

Is asthma genetic?

There's a genetic predisposition to asthma, so you're more likely to get it if it's in your family. But we haven't identified the actual gene that causes it.

When do I see a doctor if I suspect my child has asthma?

As soon as possible, because asthma is one of the leading pulmonary causes of death in children. Bring your child to a pulmonologist and an allergist.

Is there a typical age when children usually develop asthma?

No. You can develop asthma at any age.

Once you've got asthma, is it something that you have forever, or can you outgrow it?

You can outgrow it. And I believe you can cure it with a nutritional program, which is why I wrote *The Allergy and Asthma Cure: A Complete 8-Step Nutritional Program*.

How does one outgrow asthma?

The belief is that you outgrow the sensitivity to what triggers asthma, and/or your bronchi and the lining of your mucus membranes actually grow and mature, so they learn how to tolerate and deal with the outside assault on your body.

Can you develop asthma as an adult even if you didn't have it as a child?

Yes.

How can I use food to help reduce my child's allergies and asthma symptoms?

Asthma is tricky, but there are some things you can do. Get him off all yeast, which causes inflammation in the body. This is bad for any inflammatory disease such as asthma. Yeast can also cause allergies and suppresses the immune system, so if you're going to give your child bread, make sure it says "yeast-free" on the label. Also, remove the following from your child's diet: sugar, foods that are white and processed, fermented foods, vinegar, cheese, smoked meats and fish, and mushrooms. Also, limit fruit juices and milk. The sooner you start, the better off your children will be, because then eating this way will be normal for them.

Chapter 2

Prep for Your Child's Nutritional Success

I believe the old saying that "you are what you eat." I have seen way too many friends and family members get sick or die from heart disease, diabetes, cancer, etc., because of poor diet and nutrition. I feel that as parents and adults, it is our responsibility to make sure our kids are eating foods that are good for them. Eating right has to become a priority! We must take the time to cook fresh, healthy meals for our children and we have to be examples for our kids, too. They learn by watching us. I take pride in taking care of myself and my family! I do everything I can to make sure my children are getting a healthy start in life.

—Laila Ali, mother of two

Here's what I tell my children: "Don't make food your best friend. If you're extra happy or really sad, don't turn to that cupcake." With kids, we never know which lessons are absorbed and which aren't—that is, until they give us our own words right back to us. This happened to me one beautiful summer day when I was eating a bowl of sorbet and loving it so much that I barely looked up from the bowl.

"Mommy," said my then-eight-year-old daughter, Arianna. "It's okay to like that sorbet, but don't make it your best friend." This may seem like an insignificant moment, but for my family it's a symbol of how far we have come, a symbol of a happier, healthier time at the end of a long journey that changed life as I knew it and set me on a path I couldn't have predicted.

I thought my turning point in terms of my family's health was that heart-wrenching moment when I saw Addison lying on the bathroom floor. Little did I know that a second turning point would push me even further. It happened when Addison was three years old and became ill with a deadly bacterial infection that attacked his intestines. He woke up in the middle of the night with diarrhea. I thought it was a little stomach bug, similar to the one my daughter had had a few days earlier. But his was much worse. The next morning, he had diarrhea again, and again, and again. It didn't stop. My little boy was doubled over in pain, clutching his abdomen, and begging me to help his tummy stop hurting. I took a look at his stool and saw what I thought might be blood. It wasn't bright red blood and there wasn't a lot, but my intuition told me that something just didn't look right.

I called the pediatrician. "I think there's blood in Addison's stool. Can you test it?"

"For what?" she asked.

"Whatever you can!"

"Okay, but it takes four days to get bacteria test results back," she said.

"Fine."

"Then bring him in."

As soon as I hung up the phone, I took Addison to her office. By the time we got there, the diarrhea was coming every few minutes.

"He's dehydrated," the pediatrician said when she saw Addison; his skin was a dull color and his lips were dry and cracked. "Go to the hospital to get him hydrated. They won't keep your baby; they'll just do an IV to ward off further dehydration and you'll be home in no time."

I trust my pediatrician immensely, so I headed to the hospital thinking that Addison would get the IV and we'd be home by dinner. But things did not go as planned.

After a few minutes of observing Addison, and seeing how often he had to use the potty, the ER doctors were worried. An IV was not going to solve the problems they thought he had. In what seemed like minutes, they were doing an ultrasound, then a barium enema. When this didn't work, a red-haired doctor pulled me over.

"This is serious," he said. "We've got to do emergency surgery."

Emergency surgery? *I've just come to hydrate my child and now you're going to cut him open? Is this a joke? Am I being punked?* My stomach lurched and I felt as if I were going to throw up. My heart was racing, and the sweat was pouring out of me along with the tears. My hands were shaking so much that I had trouble pressing the buttons on my cell phone to call my husband. When he answered, I could barely form a coherent sentence.

"Emergency surgery. Addison. Surgery," I said.

"I'm coming. Don't let them do anything till I get there," he said.

When my husband raced into the ER, I was still holding the consent forms the doctors needed. "I can't sign these. I can't do this," I cried. I was devastated and confused. I had never in my life felt such a loss of control.

"We have to. He's sick and the doctors say this will help," my husband said.

I pushed the papers toward him. "Then you sign them. I can't."

The next thing I knew, my husband and I were being ushered into a sterile room and were putting on white scrubs. We were covered from head to toe in what looked like space suits when we went into the operating room to see Addison one last time before the surgery. He looked so small lying in the center of the operating table. I held him one last time, the lump in my throat so huge I could barely breathe. Even more heartbreaking was that Addison was too sick to protest. He was too sick to say, "Don't leave me here." He was too sick to say, "I love you." He said nothing. Absolutely nothing. I think he knew that he was so sick that this surgery was important.

Even today, a few years later, I can't think about leaving my son, my baby, in that operating room without feeling a sick sensation in the pit of my stomach and tears welling up in my eyes. There is nothing that can describe that feeling of saying good-bye to your child, knowing that when you leave, the doctors are going to cut him open.

The next hour or so was a blur, though I do remember being introduced to the person who would be performing the surgery, a female pediatric surgeon. I wanted to know who was going to touch my child, and I was relieved it was a woman. In the midst of the chaos swirling around me, I could barely speak, but I did manage to ask her, "Do you have children?" "Yes," she said. That gave me a small bit of comfort, because I knew that my tears meant something to her. She didn't see me as just another hysterical mother. She didn't think I was overreacting. She had the life of my baby in her hands and she knew what that meant.

After that, I sat huddled in the waiting room with my husband, my sister, and our pediatrician, hugging them and sobbing loudly. I didn't care who saw or heard me.

Before the surgery we'd been given all the worst-case scenarios about what they might find: "We may have to cut his intestines," "He may need a colostomy bag to use the bathroom after this," "It could be his rectum," "Maybe it's his kidneys"—the list went on and on.

Finally, he was in recovery and the doctors said we could go to him. I was not prepared for what I saw. My little three-year-old was curled up in a fetal position, a tiny ball in the midst of rumpled sheets, with tubes coming out of his arms. He was out of it, totally out of it.

"Addison. Addison," I said softly, but he didn't move.

"Why isn't he responding?" I said out loud.

"He's on morphine," one nurse replied.

"Morphine? Morphine?" Shock waves ran through my body. "Take him off of that now!" Immediately, he was taken off of it. The night nurse said the morphine was to help him with any pain. But just hours earlier the doctors had assured me that "kids are resilient," "they can tolerate pain," and "they bounce back in no time." If that was the case, why was morphine being pumped through my child's veins?

All I wanted to do was scoop him up and carry him home, but I was not even able to hold him. The pain of seeing my son curled up and drugged cut through me like a knife. On top of this, I was distraught knowing that my then-six-year-old daughter was at home feeling neglected and confused.

After Addison's surgery, the doctors were relieved. Not because they'd found something (they hadn't), but because they felt as if they'd *done* something. Still, they were puzzled when he wasn't better the next morning. Before the surgery, they had told me, "Tomorrow your son will be up and walking around. He'll be back to his old self. It'll be like he never had surgery. That's just how kids are." Not my kid. Tomorrow came, and he was still sick as a dog. He still had diarrhea. He was not eating or drinking, and he still had tubes coming out of his arms. He was lethargic, lying in a bed with metal bars that came up so high it looked like a jail cell. And he was not getting better. I kept asking the doctors questions, but they just looked at me with blank faces. They had no answers for me.

Finally, infectious disease doctors came into the room.

"The stool test came back and your son has an infection from a deadly strain of bacteria," one doctor told me. Though there was nothing they could do for this infection, they needed to keep him in the hospital to make sure the infection didn't spread.

The next few days were an emotional roller coaster ride. One day I was told the infection had hit his kidneys. The next day I was told he might need a kidney transplant and dialysis—possibly for the rest of his life. They continued taking blood and urine, and poking and prodding Addison's weary body. After a few days, his normally lean frame looked even thinner. His tiny cheeks looked sunken in. I thought, *How much more can his little body take?*

Test after test revealed that the doctors' worst-case scenarios had not come true. Still, the doctors kept saying that there was nothing they could do to help. When I called the pediatrician, she suggested giving Addison acidophilus, which is one of the live, "good" bacteria that can offset the impact of bad bacteria in the digestive tract; it's also called probiotics. Acidophilus is important to take when you're on an antibiotic, because antibiotics can remove good bacteria from the body *along with the bad*, the pediatrician explained. I'd actually heard of this good bacteria before and even had it in my house, but I hadn't given it to my kids more than once every few months. Knowing its benefits and trusting my pediatrician implicitly, I decided to follow her advice. But for some reason I felt I should consult the red-haired doctor who had been caring for Addison in the hospital.

"Can I give my son acidophilus?" I asked him.

"I don't know anything about it," he replied. "So you'd better not." He brushed me off so casually and didn't even consider my words or seem to care what I was saying.

I was fuming. *Why am I asking him?* I thought. Then I followed my instincts and loaded Addison up on acidophilus anyway, thanks to our wonderful and very aware pediatrician, Dr. Barbara Landreth.

Though I knew little about nutrition, and didn't Google things as much back then as I do today, I spent the next days trying to figure out which foods were gentle on the digestive system, such as clear, broth-based soups, and which foods would provide a lot of nutrients, such as sweet potatoes.

For the rest of Addison's stay at the hospital, my mother and I took turns going back and forth to the apartment to cook fresh food to bring to the hospital for him. It sounds crazy that you'd have to bring healthy food to a hospital, but even crazier was what they were feeding my son. He'd gone almost a week without eating anything and had just had stomach surgery, yet the first meal they gave him was sugar in various forms: white bread, apple juice, and ice cream. Their mentality was, *He's a kid. Let's pacify him with something sweet.* Perhaps that would have been okay if he'd just had his tonsils taken out or had a broken arm, but he had just had stomach surgery! His digestive system hadn't had to break down food in days. I'm certainly not a doctor, but even I know that after a week of not eating, you have to go easy on your stomach. You don't load up on sugar and fat. Later, even when they were getting ready to release Addison from the hospital, the doctors didn't even make any suggestions about his diet.

That hospital experience was several years ago, but the strong emotions I experienced during that week still hurt, and the memory still stings. To this day, we don't know the cause of my son's bacterial infection. For that I am thankful. Yes, *thankful.* If I'd been able to pinpoint the cause of that infection—bad meat or a swimming pool, for example—I would simply have removed that cause from Addison's life and continued on as before. The unknown, however, left a lot more room for change. When Addison was diagnosed with asthma and food allergies a year earlier, I had made subtle changes, but they were not enough. Now I had to do more.

As terrifying as it was, Addison's bacterial infection presented me with an opportunity. It made me more open to everything. It made me say, "Enough is enough." I was done following the traditional route and trusting other people's opinions rather than my own maternal instincts. I realized that I had to find my own answers. It was time to listen, really listen, to that little voice inside of me, urging me to pay attention. I knew the ability to help my son—to help my entire family—resided within me; it was just a matter of letting it out.

Because the bacterial infection had likely been connected to food, yet I didn't know which food, I decided that it was time to focus on our diets. (When I use the word *diet*, I am not talking about anything related to losing weight; I am referring to "a way of eating"). Our eating habits as we knew them were over. It was time to make some changes. Real changes.

Now, what I did, and what you can do, doesn't mean a drastic or total life overhaul. You don't have to detox your entire house or turn your diet upside down. Instead, you can take small, very simple actions. Maybe one or two things are all you need, or maybe they'll be the beginning of a longer journey. Either way, this is a process, and something you can eventually incorporate into your life and learn to embrace.

Stay positive and open-minded. Get inspired and excited! We are purging. We are getting rid of the unhealthy. It's like the cluttered closet you are afraid to tackle. Go in there! Because once you do, even if you clean off just one little shelf, you'll feel better and more confident. Encourage yourself. That's what I had to do. I didn't just all of a sudden have the necessary energy and motivation. No. I had to push myself and push past the doubt. I had to tell myself, *I can do this.*

We all live busy lives. We're overscheduled and constantly going, going, going. But I stopped thinking about how long any of the steps might take or what other options I had, and I made the changes a priority. Something else can always get in the way, so we really do have to prioritize. If I can do it, I know you can, too.

Come with me. We'll work together. Let's get started.

Clean Out Your Cupboards

Because I had no idea where my son had picked up that deadly strain of bacteria, I viewed everything in my kitchen as a possible culprit. During that period, ours was a typical American kitchen, filled with foods that gave my family the quick meals we needed. I was a busy mother of two, running around caring for my children on my own during the day and fulfilling the needs of a husband who was in the entertainment business at night. Like most busy moms, I thought that I didn't have time to cook fresh foods for every meal. Once we got home from the hospital, though, I knew that this needed to change, so I headed for the kitchen. I pushed up my sleeves and flung open the cabinets. Then I started looking, really looking, at what I'd been feeding my family.

READ THE LABEL

When my kids were really young, I didn't even consider reading an ingredient list. Then prior to my son's being hospitalized, when Dr. Pescatore made me aware of my children's food sensitivities and allergies, I started reading labels. But even then, I looked for only the ingredients we were allergic to. After that hospital experience, however, I started reading the labels more carefully. I looked at the ingredient lists and all the tiny words on the back of every food package. There were so many ingredients whose names I was not able to pronounce, and I didn't know what many of them were.

- **Look It Up.** If there was something I didn't understand or was unable to pronounce, I looked it up. (I still try to do this today.) It takes only seconds, and you'd be surprised how much things such as simple candy bars, chewing gum, or mints contain ingredients that are linked to cancer and other illnesses. Most of the time those long, confusing words are chemicals of some sort. Although some foods come with a good flavor, that flavor may be enhanced by a chemical, which later on may have a side effect. I'm not saying that occasionally eating foods like this is a problem. But we don't know the impact of eating a potentially disease-causing ingredient over a long period of time. Just being aware of what's in your food is important.
- **Note the Order.** The ingredients are listed in descending order, from those that are most prevalent in the food to those that appear in the smallest quantities. This is important to know, because if the

healthiest ingredients appear at the end of an ingredient list, and those such as fructose and sucrose appear at the beginning, that food may not be as healthy as we thought it was.

- **Beware of "Healthy" Foods.** Sometimes even "healthy" foods, such as flake cereals with no added sugar, contain dyes and chemicals. Then there are all the juices that actually don't have much real fruit in them, and the sports drinks (which we kept on hand if anyone in the family needed electrolytes), which are really just liquid sugar.

- **Check the Expiration Date.** I also looked at the foods' expiration dates. If the date had passed, I discarded the item. After all, the expiration date is there for a reason. Most of my canned foods had plenty of time left—years, in fact. But that got me thinking. *What chemicals are in those cans to make that food, such as chicken or vegetables in soup, last so long? What exactly is in there to make that food "fresh,"* *as the label claims?* (To me, a "fresh" food would be one that's alive. Alive meaning that it is not prepackaged and nothing is in it to add shelf life to its package.) I put the food I could donate in a box, and tossed the rest. (Yes, I felt guilty about donating foods that I no longer felt comfortable feeding to my children, but I knew there were people in shelters who were better off having some food than no food at all. It is hard to waste food knowing that someone, somewhere, may have only this to eat for their entire day.)

Detox Your Refrigerator

Next, I opened the freezer and refrigerator and threw out almost everything. Now, not all that food was unhealthy, but because I didn't know where Addison's bacterial infection had come from, I felt that everything had to go in order for us to have a fresh start. Out went the turkey burgers, beef burgers, chicken nuggets, and lamb. I started looking at everything differently. *Was that turkey responsible for Addison's illness? Or was it the beef? Maybe it was the chicken?* I had no answers. Everything became a guessing game. But this wasn't a game; it was life or death.

As I did with the food in my cupboards, I began paying attention to the labels (the meaning of the ingredients, the order of ingredients, and the expiration dates). Yes, chicken nuggets shaped like animals were cute and possibly more appealing to my kids, but their ingredients list was scary. (Today, I know there are frozen chicken nuggets that are considered decent for us, but during that period they had not yet made it into our house.) I started looking at each food and asking myself, *Are there really any vitamins in this? How is this food helping my kids?* I realized how much of my food was man-made (meaning dry and packaged), as opposed to coming from nature (meaning straight from the ground). There was colored yogurt in tubes, cheese made into sticks, and other foods designed to entice children with their bright colors, funny shapes, and silly names (and hard-to-pronounce ingredients!) right in my own refrigerator. There's nothing wrong with serving your kids these foods—on special occasions. But I had been doing it every day, or at least too often than was good for them. I had also bought into the advertising-induced fantasy that these foods were "cool." Like a lot of moms, I *wanted* my kids to be hip. When Arianna pulled out her snack at school, I *wanted* her to have the cute, colorful foods that the other kids had.

Go Beneath the Surface

Thinking about what my kids had been eating made me realize that I had been feeding them certain foods for reasons that had nothing to do with nutrition. Things such as white bread, Tater Tots, and squeezable cheese were favorite foods of mine when I was my kids' ages. Eating them as an adult brought back the warm feelings from my childhood, feelings that I thought I was passing on to my babies. For example, I used to give them turkey sandwiches on white bread because it brought back childhood memories of making turkey sandwiches on Wonder bread. This was a food my mom never bought for us, but having it at a friend's house had always been heaven. I thought that making foods such as these for my kids meant sharing my warm memories and emotions with them. But when I actually looked at the big picture, I realized that by reliving a good memory, I was creating bad habits for my kids.

Shop Smarter

CHECK OUT YOUR LOCAL HEALTH FOOD STORE

The grocery store became my religion, but I stopped shopping for most things in the regular grocery store and bought more items at the health food store. Even though that was just three years ago, things seem to have changed so much in terms of health food at supermarkets. Now you can actually find some organic foods and healthy selections in many well-known supermarket chains and at big-box stores, so you don't always have to be on the hunt for a local health food store. And remember: just because you're in the health food store doesn't mean everything there is "healthy" or right for your family. You still have to read the labels, and then decide what is healthy.

TAKE YOUR TIME

I also had to change *how* I shopped. Instead of rushing into the store and buying the same old foods, I had to start browsing the aisles, reading labels, and taking more notice of what was around me. No, I did not have two free hours to shop—especially at that time, when only one of my kids was in school full-time. (And I still don't have two free hours.) But those first few weeks after Addison got home from the hospital, I had to take a little extra time. I didn't have anyone to walk me through the store, no grocery store tour guide greeting me and teaching me how to read a label. I was schooling myself, so I had to make the sacrifice and take the time. It was a priority. I had to learn what foods were out there, what the store had to offer. Soon enough, shopping became as quick and easy as it had been before. So that initial investment in my time was worth it. For example, to get an item containing vitamin C, I used to grab orange juice in a carton from the refrigerated aisle. Now I grab kale from the produce aisle and blueberry juice in a glass jar from the dry foods aisle.

BUY FRESH

During that first year after my son was in the hospital, I focused on buying a lot more fresh foods and went for frozen foods over canned, because foods that are frozen are usually frozen fresh, and contain fewer preservatives.

CHECK OUT YOUR LOCAL FARMERS' MARKET

Farmers' markets are a great place to get fresh fruits and vegetables. Typically these foods come from nearby farms and gardens, instead of traveling from other states and countries. This shorter travel time from the farm or garden to your table can mean that the foods contain more nutrients, were handled by fewer people, and are less likely to have been damaged or abused along the way. Also, local food tends to be in season, and as you'll read a little later on, eating in-season foods is important.

Be Open to New Information

As I said earlier, the period of Addison's illness was one in which my eyes and ears were wide open. I read a lot. I listened a lot. I asked a lot of questions. I was already past high school, so I knew there was no such thing as a dumb question. (Nor did I care if anyone thought my questions were dumb.) I didn't take every piece of advice I was given; sometimes I didn't take any. But I still listened with an open mind, letting go of preconceptions and expectations.

Today the resources we have for information on food are endless. You can go to a library or bookstore, search the Internet, or take a class. If you don't have a computer, try asking a friend or librarian to Google the information for you. We are the voice for our children, so until they're able to look for information themselves on how to live healthier, and fully understand it, we've got to do it for them. It is one of our responsibilities as moms, dads, and caregivers. And I promise that it's not as overwhelming as it sounds. I spent a lot of time asking questions of the people who ran my local health food store. (One piece of advice I ended up following, and still do today, was to give my kids cod-liver oil because it has omega-3 fatty acids and vitamins A, D3, and E.)

Believe in Yourself

It wasn't easy for me to go on this journey, especially because I was on it alone. I had no friends eating the way we were, my mother thought I was crazy, and my husband sometimes gave me "the look." But something inside me, my inner voice, told me that this was the right road to take. Even today if my son says, "My ear hurts. I think I need onion," my husband looks at me like "Oh Lord." But I don't care, because I know it works. I've read, I've listened, and I've experimented. I've tried this stuff, and there *are* results. I can't say it will work for every single person every time. But it can't hurt to try.

ANSWERS FROM ERICA'S EXPERT

Barbara Landreth, MD, practices Western medicine but has always been supportive when I wanted to take an alternative route. She is an assistant attending pediatrician at New York–Presbyterian Hospital/Weill Cornell Medical Center and an assistant attending pediatrician at Lenox Hill Hospital. In addition, she is a clinical instructor in pediatrics at Weill Cornell Medical College. She's been my children's pediatrician since I was pregnant with Arianna. My husband and I were interviewing pediatricians and we immediately connected with her and loved her. As soon as Arianna was born, Dr. Landreth came to the hospital to meet her and give her a routine new birth checkup. She was so patient, kind, gentle, and supportive. She showed me how to get Arianna to latch on while nursing and helped me settle in with my precious baby while in the hospital room. Not only did she provide this loving care with my firstborn, but my secondborn, Addison, received the same care and concern. Dr. Landreth is also the mother of two boys, ages twenty-four and twenty-eight.

Healthy Eating

What are the worst foods and ingredients for children to eat?

The worst foods and ingredients in your child's diet are those to which your child reacts immediately with symptoms such as irritability, vomiting, diarrhea, rash, and hyperactivity. The most common ones are sugar, corn syrup, artificial sweeteners, dyes, eggs, fish, nuts, milk, soy, wheat, citrus, and tomato. Besides these, any "low fat" foods or milk, because they actually promote hunger because they don't satisfy our appetites, they have artificial ingredients, and fat is necessary in our diets. Due to the increase of autism in the United States, I would also not recommend any baby formula or prepared baby food with the added synthetic DHA or ARA.

What one thing do you wish parents understood about feeding their children?

Parents need to learn how to design healthy diets for themselves. They are the models for their children. If they don't snack, if they prepare healthy meals for themselves and sit down together at the dinner table without TV and laptops to distract them, they will have all the fundamentals about feeding their children.

It seems as if children today are always snacking—in strollers, midway through soccer games, walking home from school, etc. What are your thoughts on snacking?

Children are taught habits from the day they are born. Allowing a baby to breast-feed every hour or a toddler to eat pretzels in his stroller or a child to eat a hot dog on his way home from school is allowing "snacking." Parents should realize that their children's soothing or happiness cannot be related to food. Taking the baby out for a walk, giving the toddler a book, and letting a child run in the playground can be lifesaving for them as teenagers and adults; they will learn the habit of not using food as comfort. Parents should not introduce snacks to their children, as children do not need to eat between meals. Nibbling all day long can start lifelong weight problems. Plus, constantly snacking makes you hungry.

We know childhood obesity is an epidemic. What are some things moms and dads can do to help prevent this in their children?

Childhood obesity can be prevented with parents learning how to eat well and being role models for their children, sitting down with the family at least three times a week to a home-cooked dinner with conversation and no distractions, and spending twenty minutes a day playing outdoors and breaking a sweat with their children.

If a family has not been eating healthy foods, but you want to change that, what are some suggestions?

I recommend the book *The Healthy Way to Changing Carbs: Weight Control and Weight Loss for Families with Kids*, by Arnold Slyper, MD, and its companion website, www.eatforhealth.org.

Are artificial sweeteners really bad for children?

The FDA-approved artificial sweeteners are saccharin (Sweet'N Low), aspartame (NutraSweet, Equal, SugarTwin), acesulfame potassium, neotame, and sucralose (Splenda). All these are also used in many foods and beverages, so read the labels. None of the manufacturers of these products have conducted long-term studies, and the Food and Drug Administration is not requiring them to do so. Until such studies are presented to us, it would be best for pregnant women and children to avoid these sweeteners. All have been reported to have side effects such as headache, fatigue, rash, and depression. Since the 1970s, many studies have also shown that these products can actually *cause* weight gain. The possible reason for this is that artificial sugars, much like low-fat milk, can increase caloric cravings. For an informed review of artificial sweeteners, please refer to www.medicinenet.com/artificial_sweeteners/article.htm.

When it comes to babies, what's the best way to start giving them solid foods?

I have studied many papers and have to agree with the latest American Academy of Pediatrics Policy Statement (2008). According to this and to Scott Sicherer, an author and a doctor in Hugh Sampson's practice, there is no reason to restrict any food. Here are some pertinent sentences from this policy statement: "Although no solid foods should be introduced before four to six months of age, there is no current convincing evidence that delaying their introduction beyond this period has a significant protective effect on the development of atopic disease regardless of whether infants are fed cow milk protein formula or human milk. This includes delaying the introduction of foods that are considered to be highly allergenic, such as fish, eggs, and foods containing peanut protein. For infants after four to six months of age, there are insufficient data to support a protective effect of any dietary intervention for the development of atopic disease."

Five Months

Week 1:

Days 1–4: Breakfast of rice cereal as follows:

First day: 1 tablespoon rice cereal, plus mother's milk/formula

Second day: 2 tablespoons, plus mother's milk/formula

Third day: 3 tablespoons, plus mother's milk/formula

Each day thereafter: 4 tablespoons, plus mother's milk/formula

Days 5–7: Add dinner of rice cereal (4 tablespoons)

Week 2:

Days 1–4: Breakfast of oatmeal cereal (4 tablespoons); dinner of rice cereal

Days 5–7: Breakfast and dinner of oatmeal cereal (4 tablespoons)

Week 3:

Days 1–4: Breakfast of multigrain cereal (4 tablespoons); dinner of oatmeal cereal

Days 5–7: Breakfast and dinner of multigrain cereal

Week 4:

Days 1–4: Breakfast and dinner of rice, oatmeal, *or* multigrain cereal

Days 5–7: Breakfast and dinner—Add 2 tablespoons pureed, cooked fruit (applesauce *or* pears *or* peaches *or* prunes) *or* ½ mashed banana to cereal.

Add only one new food at a time. Feed three to five days in a row before starting another new food. In the meantime, foods already given may be repeated.

Do parents need to give their children vitamin supplements?

Vitamin supplements are recommended by the American Academy of Pediatrics. Until a child is drinking 32 ounces of vitamin-fortified formula, the child needs to take supplemental vitamin D, which is not delivered in breast milk and is not adequately delivered in lesser amounts of formula. Any liquid infant vitamin preparation with vitamins A, D, and C with 400 IU of vitamin D per dropperful is recommended. (A popular brand is Tri-Vi-Sol.) One

---

STARTING FOODS

6 months: ADD Lunch 4 hours after Breakfast.

Add only one new food at a time. Have children's diphenhydramine HCl (Benadryl) handy when starting new foods. Feed any new food three to five days in a row before starting another new food. In the meantime, foods already given may be repeated.

BREAKFAST
cereal
fruit

LUNCH
white starch (pasta, rice, potato)
colored vegetable
fruit

DINNER
cereal
fruit

At 7 months, ADD:
cooked egg yolk 3x a week
bagel
toast
At 9 months:
1 whole egg 3x a week

At 7 months, ADD:
plain meats & proteins

At 9 months:
ADD fish to meat & protein choices

At 7 months, ADD:
yogurt
cottage cheese
vanilla ice cream

BABY CEREAL	VEGETABLES	FRUITS	PLAIN MEATS & PROTEINS	INFANT JUICES (Only for constipation)
Portion 4 tablespoons per serving (+ fruit)	2.5 oz Jar Portions 1st day: ⅓ jar 2nd day: ⅓ jar 3rd day: ⅓ jar Thereafter: 1 jar	2.5 oz Jar Portions 1 jar	2.5 oz Jar Portions 1st day: ⅓ jar 2nd day: ⅓ jar 3rd day: ⅓ jar Thereafter: ⅓ - 1 jar	Portion 2 fl oz + 2 fl oz of water once a day
☐ RICE CEREAL ☐ OATMEAL ☐ MULTI-GRAIN CEREAL ☐ BARLEY CEREAL > 6 mo	☐ CARROTS ☐ PEAS ☐ SQUASH ☐ GREEN BEANS ☐ SWEET POTATOES	☐ APPLESAUCE ☐ PEARS ☐ PEACHES ☐ BANANAS ☐ PRUNES	☐ LAMB ☐ CHICKEN ☐ BEEF ☐ HAM ☐ TURKEY ☐ VEAL ☐ BEANS ☐ TOFU ☐ SPINACH	☐ PEAR JUICE ☐ WHITE GRAPE JUICE ☐ PRUNE JUICE

ADDITIONAL INSTRUCTIONS
Do not try mixed foods until single foods are tolerated well.
NO HONEY until 1ˢᵗ birthday.

---

dropperful a day should be given until the child is drinking 32 ounces of formula a day.

Do the candylike vitamins—such as gummy bears and chewable candies—really have vitamins in them?

Older children need vitamin D in their diets, too. If they are not drinking at least two 8-ounce portions of milk a day they will need supplemental vitamin D in liquid or chewable form. In addition, the American Academy of Pediatrics recommends vitamins with iron. Gummy-type vitamins do not have iron, and if they advertise that they do, the iron is not well absorbed in this form. So it is best to give a chewable multivitamin plus iron with at least 400 IU of vitamin D or an equivalent liquid vitamin plus iron on a daily basis.

Is it healthy for a child to be a vegetarian?

It may be healthy for a child to be a vegetarian as long as the child is given supplemental vitamins with iron. If the child is not drinking milk, vitamin D should also be in his daily iron vitamin. A child on a normal diet should have his blood tested at age nine months for the following:

- Complete blood count, which includes the white blood count (white blood cells fight infection); red blood count (red blood cells deliver oxygen); and platelet blood count (platelets are the cells needed in blood clotting)
- Lead level to measure any toxic amounts
- Iron level, as iron is needed for red blood cells to deliver oxygen

A child on a vegan diet should have this blood test repeated at age fifteen months and thirty months, with the addition of measurements for vitamin D and vitamin B_{12} levels.

If a child is a vegetarian, how can she get protein and the other nutrients she needs to grow properly?

Milk is a perfect food, especially if it is whole milk and comes from grass-fed cows. Cows are meant to eat grass, not grain. Some organic milk is from grain-fed cows, who do not produce omega-3s as a result. If a child cannot tolerate milk, the rice milks and soy milks that are available with supplemental calcium and vitamin D are sufficient.

Are frozen foods okay for kids to eat? Are they as healthy as fresh?

Frozen or canned (in non-BPA containers) vegetables can be as healthy as, or healthier than, fresh vegetables because they are generally picked when their nutrient content is at its peak and frozen or canned. Beware of any salt added to such vegetables. Many "fresh" vegetables in the supermarket may have lost their nutritive value, and when parents cook vegetables too long or in too much water it can destroy their nutrients. So if you cannot buy fresh, ripe, local, in-season vegetables, or if there are any doubts about the freshness of the vegetables in the market, or about how to cook them properly, frozen or canned (in non-BPA containers) vegetables are a healthier bet, especially if one follows the cooking directions and chooses the "no salt added" varieties.

How do I know if my child's stomachache is food related or viral related?

A virus will give bad cramping, relieved by vomiting and/or diarrhea, and will continue with diarrhea. These symptoms may last over a period of hours or days. A bacterial infection will give the same symptoms, but the diarrhea will be bloody, because bacteria harm the wall of the blood-lined intestine and these symptoms may also last for hours or days. Fever is more common with bacterial bellyaches. A food may give bloating, discomfort, possible mild cramping, and diarrhea within a half hour of being eaten. These symptoms will not continue once the diarrhea has occurred. If a child is seriously allergic to a food, these symptoms may be accompanied by swelling of the lips and/or eyelids, coughing, difficulty swallowing, hives, and itchiness. If this occurs, the parent must call 911, as it could be life threatening.

What do you see most often in your office that could be ameliorated by one simple change?

Children two to five years of age are already overweight or obese. An average of 24.5 percent of American children are obese or overweight. Overweight and obese status during this period in childhood has been found to persist into adolescence and adulthood. Establishing healthy eating habits and engaging in routine physical activity that includes both parents and children earlier in childhood will improve the parents' health and the health of their children. The Centers for Disease Control and Prevention has recommended that children and adolescents participate in at least 60 minutes of moderate-intensity exercise each day and that adults participate in at least 2.5 hours of moderate-intensity physical activity and 2 hours of strength training every week.[*]

What is one thing that parents seem to worry about most but that really isn't an issue?

Fever in a child is what parents fear most. They do not have to fear fever, as it is a sign that the child is actively fighting an infection. A fever in a child is any body temperature over 100.5 degrees Fahrenheit or 38 degrees Celsius, ideally taken with a rectal thermometer, especially for children under

---

[*] U.S. Department of Health and Human Services, Physical Activity Guidelines for Americans, available at: www.health.gov/paguidelines/, accessed July 20, 2009.

the age of 2. Fever, unless over 105 degrees, is normal, and expected in the course of a child's early years. Viral infections tend to affect the entire body and give higher temperatures than bacterial infections that affect one part—for example, the ear, the throat, the bladder. Fever control is indicated only to make the child feel better, so the child will eat, drink, and sleep.

For a child over 6 months of age, ibuprofen (Children's Advil or Motrin) is recommended at a dose of 100 milligrams per 20 pounds of body weight every 6 hours while the child is awake. For example, a 20-pound child would need 100 milligrams (1 teaspoon) every 6 hours. A 30-pound child would need 150 milligrams (1 ½ teaspoons) every 6 hours, and a 60-pound child would need 300 milligrams (3 teaspoons) every 6 hours.

For a child under 6 months of age, acetaminophen (Children's Tylenol) is recommended at a dose of 160 milligrams per 20 pounds of body weight every 4 hours while the child is awake. For example, a 20-pound child would need 160 milligrams (1 teaspoon) every 4 hours. A 10-pound child would need 80 milligrams (½ teaspoon) every 4 hours while awake, and a 15-pound child would need 120 milligrams (¾ teaspoon) every 4 hours while awake.

The parents must call their doctor or go to the emergency room if any one of the following occurs after they've given the medicines:

- The child is extremely cranky, *or*
- The child has developed other symptoms, such as vomiting, rash, or unusual drowsiness, *or*
- The child's fever continues to go up, *or*
- The child, under the age of two years, continues to have a fever for a full three days. (Under the age of two *months*, any fever in a child is an emergency and *no* medicines should be given until the child sees a doctor or goes to the emergency room.)

Do you think that the foods kids eat can affect their behavior?

"We are what we eat" in the sense that ours and our children's health, vitality, behavior, and misbehavior are affected by our food choices. If you find that your child is unusually sleepy after having meals of bagels, cereal, pasta, pizza, or any wheat-containing product, you might consider that he has a condition known as *celiac disease,* especially if he has exhibited any growth slowdown. This is a sensitivity to gluten, which is found in wheat, barley, rye, and possibly oats. Consult with your doctor about your suspicion as a simple blood test can suggest gluten sensitivity. Snack foods that end in the letter O (such as Cheetos, Doritos, Oreos, Fritos, Tostitos, etc.) may also be culprits in your child's sleepiness, tiredness, dizziness, irritability, or depression after eating. These foods have high fat and high sugar content and lack any nutritional value. Withdrawal symptoms after excess fat and sugar include sleepiness, which is caused by serotonin, a neurochemical produced in the body in response to high fat and sugar consumption. Watch your children for clues that poor food choices are being made.

We know that there are some vaccines that have components that some children may be allergic to. So, if there's a history of food allergies in a family, do you recommend waiting to vaccinate a child until you know whether that child has food allergies?

A life-threatening food allergy to egg is a contraindication to your child's receiving any flu vaccine (influenza A and B) or any yellow fever vaccine. Otherwise, all other vaccines are safe for children who have food allergies.

Why is calcium so important?

It's all about your child's bone density. If your child doesn't get enough calcium, there can be problems—especially with girls. They need as much calcium as possible before age twenty-one, because calcium stores from childhood prevent brittle bone disease later in life. So add more broccoli and yogurt to your child's diet.

What else is important for your child's health?

Focus on sleep issues. Lack of sleep compromises your child's immune system. I know many working moms don't see their children until late, so they want to keep them up, but you still have to keep bedtime issues in mind. If your child is tired, he or she won't learn as well, accept discipline, or make good choices. Exercise is also crucial. I recommend your child breaking out into a sweat for at least twenty minutes a day from exercise. At the very least, try to walk around the block after dinner. It's so important to turn off the video games and get those couch potatoes outside.

Chapter 3

Make Over Your Child's Diet

I am a big believer in whole natural foods. I read labels carefully and try to avoid foods with lots of additives and chemicals. For that reason, I tend to buy most of my food in a health food store. The cookies I buy for my kids contain no sugar, no dyes, and no preservatives. It costs a little more, but it's worth it to me in the long run.

—Bobbi Brown, mother of three

For years, I had heard friends in California talk about an incredible woman, Mina Dobic, who taught self-healing through macrobiotic living. Mina was well-known for using whole organic foods to help people prevent, manage, or cure illness. She had treated many celebrities and several friends of ours who were living with serious health conditions. But most impressive was the story of how she'd treated herself.

Twenty-four years ago, Mina was diagnosed with stage-four ovarian cancer, which had metastasized to her liver, bones, and lymphatic system. The doctors gave her just two months to live, but she healed herself with macrobiotics and is still alive and healthy today. And she still lives the macrobiotic way of life, walking the walk. (Mina Dobic's full story is featured in her book *My Beautiful Life: How I Conquered Cancer Naturally*, which has been translated into many languages.)

At the point when Addison came home from the hospital, I knew I needed to do more than just detox my kitchen and read food labels. I'm not saying that I knew macrobiotics was the answer. In fact, I knew little about it, except that the idea behind it was to use food in a healing way. We hear about food being "good" or "bad" only when it comes to weight and to conditions such as high cholesterol, heart disease, and obesity, but we don't hear enough about it being used in a medicinal way. But at that point, I was ready and willing to use the things we normally took for granted, such as grocery shopping and cooking, as medicine for my family's good health. I was also ready to open my eyes and ears in a way they had never been open before. Addison's time in the hospital was presenting me with yet another opportunity to learn.

This time I didn't want to go only to traditional doctors. I loved our traditional Western doctors—our pediatrician is one of the best, someone whom I respect, and who has always been dedicated to our family—but I had to tackle my son's health in a different way this time. Never again could I watch him suffer as I had during that week in the hospital. More important, I didn't just want him better; I wanted him healthy! I wanted to help him build up his immune system.

I called a friend in California who had told me stories about Mina and asked her to help me track down her phone number. Once I reached her, I explained our situation and offered to fly her to New York. (I used our frequent-flier miles.) She agreed, and about two weeks later she arrived at our apartment. Now, here is where a lot of people may roll their eyes, thinking they don't have the money or the time to fly in a macrobiotic guru. (It even sounds crazy to me as I write it!) Yes, it was costly and time-consuming, but it had already been costly and time-consuming to schlep back and forth to doctors' offices and follow-up visits for over a year. It had already been costly and time-consuming going repeatedly to the drugstore and paying for medication—even with health insurance. I had to look at the big picture, and that picture was telling me to find the root cause of my son's health problems, not just to deal with the symptoms as I had been doing up until then. I was also hungry and desperate to heal my son, and when you are hungry and desperate, you'll try anything.

Usually I consult with my husband before hiring anyone, because it can be costly and I want to be respectful, mindful, and considerate. After all, it's not like buying a pair of shoes or a purse. But when it came to Mina, I didn't ask. This was our son and his health. I then decided that my daughter and I would also follow what Mina suggested, because the two of us also had food allergies and health issues. Why not let us all benefit from her wisdom?

So Mina came into our home. She was very wise, aware, and an expert in her field. Her spirit was kind, gentle, caring, and so positive. Her warmth was so inviting that we embraced her easily and felt very comfortable in her presence. For such a petite woman, she came in and made some big—and I mean very big—changes. A macrobiotic diet is considered a healing diet and is known for its positive impact on cancer. But macrobiotics is also a lifestyle. Mina not only told us basically to stop eating everything we'd been eating, but she also suggested body products and types of baths we needed to take. (For example, she had me taking sitz baths with dried Japanese leaves called daikon, and my kids were taking oat bran baths.)

Macrobiotics focuses not only on what you eat, but *how* you eat it. You don't just gobble down a meal, but instead chew each bite thirty to fifty times, so it's digested better. Clearly, counting how many times I chewed, and making two small children do the same, just wasn't going to happen. So I had to take from Mina's suggestions what would work for our home—just as you should take from this book what will work for yours. Even if you can only do a few of the things outlined here, some of the way is better than none of the way. One change may make you feel so good that you try another and then another, and slowly but surely, you're transforming your life. The following are simple steps that I took that made the biggest difference.

Was it hard for me? Absolutely, but I knew that I would set the tone for my kids, so I didn't act as if it were hard, and I tried not to complain. My kids are active children who used to like going to the local restaurant for mac 'n' cheese, chicken fingers, French fries, and hot dogs—you know, the typical kid-friendly American fare—so it wasn't easy for them either. Also, using food as medicine was totally new to me, and I had no one to share the experience with; none of my friends were eating this way, and my mother thought I was crazy. She didn't think I was giving my growing children enough food. Moreover, she thought the food I was feeding them was flavorless, because macrobiotic food tastes different from the processed foods we're used to. And then there was my husband, who thought, *Here's Erica doing some hokey experiment.* Along with being a laughingstock to my friends and family, I felt like my own guinea pig. But my gut was telling me to start this journey and I was willing to deal with some tough stuff to get there.

Under Mina's guidance, we followed a strict macrobiotic diet for one year. Some people can do it for longer; some people cannot. For my family, it was challenging, because we travel often and at the time, my daughter, being the only one in school full-time, was not allowed to bring her own lunch to school and feel comfortable and supported doing so. (More on that in chapter 6, "Thriving at School.") Still, I decided to make the investment and make it work for that year, and I am grateful for it. Today, though we are by no means strict macrobiotics, I do apply some of the elements we learned during that year and those that I believe truly changed my family's health. If you or a loved one has a serious illness and you choose to try macrobiotics, look for an expert who has years of experience in this field and who has benefited from it. Reach out to people who are truly living that way and read as much about macrobiotics as you can. Then just go for it—but one day at a time. Don't say, "I can't do this for the rest of the week/month/year." Instead, focus on doing it today and today only, and before you know it, it'll become part of your life.

What I'm about to share is by no means a strict macrobiotic diet. Instead, it includes some of the elements that worked best for my family and fit most easily in our lives. At the time I was trying it for my kids, I was very much alone. Everything was trial and error. I was out there researching on my own. Now I hope I can spare you some of the running-around-like-a-chicken-with-its-head-cut-off feeling that I experienced. These are actionable steps that anyone can take to improve their health and the health of their loved ones, using products available to everyone in every city.

Cut Back on Processed Foods

One of the biggest changes you can make in your diet is to reduce how many processed foods you eat. And it's really not that hard. For example, instead of frozen, packaged chicken and frozen veggies for dinner one night, use the fresh version of one of those items. The time it takes for chicken nuggets to bake is more than enough time to take broccoli out of the fridge, cut it, and steam it.

Many moms believe that what our kids eat when they're young doesn't make a difference to their long-term health, and I admit I used to be one of them. But actually, it does matter. If a child is fed chocolate milk or sugared cereal for breakfast when he's four or five years old, he comes to expect that food each morning, develops a physical craving for sugar to start his day, and shapes his eating style to reflect those early choices. Most likely, this is a habit he'll carry with him for the rest of his life. And who formed it? We did as moms and dads, right in our own homes.

The snacks I used to give my kids included a lot of processed foods. For example, my daughter and I used to eat chips or crackers with squeezable cheese in a can. I thought it was cute and fun, and I figured, *Cheese has calcium, so there can't be anything wrong with it*. But with Mina's advice, all that changed. Our snacks became sheets of nori, rice cakes topped with applesauce, brown rice crackers, edamame, sliced carrots, hummus, seedless grapes, and fruit smoothies. (See "Really Easy Recipes Your Kids Will Love.") Although we occasionally snack on some items that are not the best for us, these healthy snacks are the ones I usually try to encourage.

Visit the Vegetable and Fruit Aisle

Before Addison's hospital stay, broccoli and frozen peas were pretty much the only vegetables my kids ate. If they had collard greens, it was at Thanksgiving or during a good old soul food dinner on a Sunday evening three to four times a year. But those greens were cooked so much that they were soggy and dark in color, and probably didn't have a vitamin left in them. Once we changed our ways, we expanded the meaning of "veggies" to include sea vegetables such as seaweed, a Japanese radish called daikon, kale, collard greens, asparagus, artichokes, edamame, and mushrooms, among other vegetables we'd never eaten before (and many we hadn't ever heard of!).

We also ate fresh vegetable soups such as onion, broccoli, carrot ginger, and lots of miso soup—all of which were very different from the high-sodium canned soups we had been used to. And boy, did we used to like that canned soup! I'd always thought the easiest thing to do was to open a can of soup and heat it in a pot. But making fresh soup is just as easy. It involves throwing veggies in a pot with water to cook and then putting the cooked veggies in a blender and pressing the Puree button. You don't even have to chop the vegetables that much or that well, because once they get soft, the blender does the rest of the work. The point is you don't have to be a gourmet chef, or a chef of any sort, to make fresh homemade soup. You just have to find ways to cook that are simple and that work for you and your family. (For more on this, see "Really Easy Recipes Your Kids Will Love.")

There were some "new" veggies on the macrobiotic diet my kids did not want to go near. For example, Mina suggested something called a "pressed salad," made with cabbage, cucumbers, and radish that have been pressed with a plate. I knew my kids had no interest in this type of salad (and I didn't make a big fuss about it), but I liked it. After all, I wanted to benefit from Mina's suggestions, too, and see the results she said I would experience, such as better skin, hair, and nails, in addition to overall better health. (And yes, I did experience some of those benefits such as clearer skin.)

Cut Back on Sugar

It's hard to pick any one thing that made the biggest difference in my family's health, but if I had to, at the top of my list would be eliminating sugar—not sweeteners, but sugar. (On a macrobiotic diet there is no white or brown sugar allowed.) It wasn't easy cutting it from our diets. After all, I had two children who still wanted their sweets, and a son whom I called my "sugar child." He wanted the stuff morning, noon, and night. (And then there were my monthly sugar cravings.) I didn't want to deprive my kids or make dessert off-limits. Besides, Mina absolutely believed in having dessert after dinner—just healthier versions. So I learned to create satisfying sweet treats that had some nutritional value. (See "Really Easy Recipes Your Kids Will Love.") I also learned what sugar actually does to your body, and was shocked to find that besides giving you energy highs followed by big crashes, it suppresses your immune system and affects every cell in your body, including your skin.

One of our favorite healthy desserts became something called Kanten, a good-for-you Japanese version of Jell-O that's not packed with preservatives or food coloring. It's made with something called agar and sea vegetables. Amazingly, my kids love it, and I'm still surprised at their excitement each time I make it today. (See recipes for Kanten in "Really Easy Recipes Your Kids Will Love.")

We also learned to appreciate the natural sugar that's in fruit—enjoying desserts such as pears with strawberry sauce—and discovered new sweeteners such as real pure maple syrup, brown rice syrup, and agave. So good-bye, brown and white sugar; hello, real alternative sweeteners (and I don't mean those sweeteners that come in little pink, yellow, and blue packets that you tear open with your teeth).

My goal was not to deprive my children, but to find ways to make the foods they ate more beneficial to their bodies. So I did some experimenting in the kitchen (and I still experiment), and as a result I have found some great ways of making healthy treats such as sugar-free, dairy-free, egg-free muffins, cupcakes, and cookies. My kids and I will also take strawberries and blueberries and make a dairy-free smoothie with rice or soy milk and non-concentrated apple juice. My kids love it, and I freeze the leftover mixture into little ice pops for later. If it's summertime or you live in a climate that's warm all year, you can do this often. Another favorite snack is Arianna's homemade granola. She learned the recipe from someone who was cooking in our home, but Arianna has perfected it, and I have to admit it is even better than mine.

What's surprising is that I used to hate cooking. I felt as if it took all day to prepare something that took just minutes to eat. The only thing I enjoyed doing in the kitchen was eating. But after hiring Mina, instead of thinking about how much work it took, I started thinking about the benefits my family was receiving. I had to learn to like cooking. And I finally did—at least a little bit. It has become like a fun science project to me, mixing things together and creating something delicious and memorable. (Not the case all the time, but most of the time!)

Change Your Drinks

I used to think that a glass of juice was what my kids needed to start their day. After all, juice is from fruit, so it must be healthy, right? Not really. Once I started paying attention, I realized that a lot of juice contains very little fruit and a lot of sugar, and much of it is concentrated, which means highly processed and most of the nutrients removed. My kids have juice occasionally now, but it's *when* they have it that matters. Right before school? Nope. At that point, sugar and chemicals aren't going to help them perform academically, concentrate, behave properly, or be able to get through their day. But on a weekend or vacation? Yes, they can have some juice, because the same academic pressure is not put on them during the weekend or on vacation as it is during a full day of school.

We also started drinking a lot more water. On a sweltering day, I will give my children cold water to cool down, but day to day, we drink our water at room temperature. Mina taught us that room temperature water is easier on the digestive system than cold. I encourage the kids to drink water by keeping a pitcher of it, and glasses, on the counter at all times. What I've found is that if it's easily available, they'll drink more than they would if the pitcher weren't out on the counter. In addition, this helps them feel more independent. (Yes, there are times when they get themselves a freezing cold glass of water, but it's not the example we set in our home.)

Before we went macrobiotic, my kids drank ginger ale and that greenish-colored sports drink. Now, on occasion, they'll have a ginger ale or a Shirley Temple if we're eating in a restaurant, traveling on an airplane, away on vacation, but rarely at home. I'm not saying you can't have a bubbly, sweet drink; just restrict how often you do. Both regular soda and those labeled "diet" are loaded with sugar, dyes, and other unhealthy ingredients. My kids love a little bubbly water with certain things added to it. So add club soda or sparkling water to any juice to dilute the sugar, or add sliced oranges or agave nectar to plain or sparkling water to sweeten it up. (See recipes on pp. 237–238.)

Avoid Foods Without Real Vitamins in Them

That's my rule of thumb, and it's a helpful one when trying to decide what to feed your kids. Does that bag of candy have real vitamins in it? No. So what's the point of giving them something filled with sugar and dye? Is it so they can be hyper? Concentrate less? Feel foggy mentally? Or is it to pacify them or be the best or coolest mommy or daddy? Better on-the-go snack options include raisins; trail mix; and carrot, blueberry, or zucchini muffins. (A donut is not a muffin.) There are many other options, such as applesauce, rice cakes with manuka honey on top, or granola.

Go Organic (When Possible)

Before I started this journey, I didn't truly know what "organic" meant or how it was different from "natural." I only saw the word *organic* showing up on a lot of food items. But I had to find out.

Many of us think "natural" means that a food comes from the earth, but that's not necessarily true. Food manufacturers' definition of "natural" is not always clear, but when it comes to the label "organic," foods grown without synthetic pesticides or petroleum-based fertilizers, there are some regulations. "Organic" also refers to how a food is produced. According to U.S. Department of Agriculture (USDA) regulations, if a product label reads, "100% organic," all the agricultural ingredients it contains are certified organic. If it reads, "organic," 95 percent of the ingredients are certified organic; and if it reads, "made with organic ingredients," at least 70 percent are certified organic.

Initially, I went organic with everything. Yes, it was expensive, but my children's health was at stake. To cut down on the cost of your grocery bill, you can be selective in which foods you buy organic and which not. My rule of thumb? If you eat the entire food, skin included, such as with an apple or a peach, try to go organic. But if it's a food that has a protective skin, such as an orange or a banana, you can skip the organic version if cost is an issue. (But rinse that skin carefully before cutting or peeling the fruit, so any chemicals or bacteria on it don't pass onto the part of the fruit you eat.)

Another way to determine what to buy organic is to find out which fruits and vegetables contain the most and least amounts of pesticide. The Environmental Working Group (EWG), a nonprofit research organization in Washington, D.C., that focuses on human health and the environment, has created a list of the twelve fruits and veggies contaminated with the most pesticides, which they call "The Dirty Dozen," and a list of the fifteen that contain the least amount of pesticides, which they call "The Clean 15." The EWG created these lists after analyzing information from almost eighty-nine thousand tests for pesticide residue collected by both the USDA and the Food and Drug Administration (FDA). (You can download both these lists or EWG's app at www.foodnews.org.)

I also suggest you choose the organic versions when buying dairy and poultry products. That's because when it comes to chicken, milk, cheese, and eggs, conventional versions may contain hormones and antibiotics. The issue with hormones is that they can cause extra growth in certain parts of the body (for example, the breasts on a young girl). The issue with antibiotics is that we are receiving an unnecessary dose of these medications. Whatever is fed to animals to eat, you are likely eating and digesting the same thing as that animal.

Over time, organic food seems to have become more readily available, and it is hoped that prices for organically grown products will go down, so they become an option for anybody who wants to eat clean, beneficial foods. After all, a luxury is flying a private plane or chartering a yacht, not eating organic or fresh, healthy foods. Caring for ourselves and our children through food should not be considered a luxury.

Eat with the Seasons

Mina introduced me to the idea of eating according to the seasons. When she first entered our home, it was fall and I had pineapples, oranges, and tomatoes in the fruit basket on my kitchen counter.

"Where are they growing pineapples or tomatoes right now during the fall season in New York?" Mina asked.

I shrugged. I had no idea. Then I thought about how high in tomatoes my kids' diets were, thanks to all the pasta sauce and ketchup they were eating.

"No wonder your daughter has eczema," Mina said. "Tomatoes are too acidic to be eaten in such high quantities, and also it is freezing cold and dry outside right now." She went on to explain that one should consume only foods that are grown locally and in season. "You need to eat foods that are thriving where you are," she said.

Though I'd never thought of this before, it made complete sense. (It also made me realize that I'd never thought much about where our food *came from*.) So we started eating local foods that were in season, such as apples and pears in the fall and peaches and tomatoes in the summer. I love pineapple, and it was hard to give it up, so if I'm ever somewhere warm and tropical, I'll have it every day.

Prepare Food in Bulk

Most people opt for takeout, prepared, or restaurant meals because they're too busy to cook. Yet convenience can have a high price tag, especially to our health. Cooking at home is typically much less expensive than going out to eat, and it certainly can be healthier. We usually eat meals prepared at home because I know where the ingredients have come from, how they've been handled, and how the food has been prepared. The way I make eating at home work for me and my schedule is that I cook in bulk. I don't have the time to cook every day, so I set aside one day to prepare food for the week. Pick whichever day works best for you—and you don't need the whole day, just a few hours. Mondays typically work best for me, because that's when I have a babysitter. That gives me time to go grocery shopping, soak my beans, clean and chop my vegetables, and make large pots of rice, beans, and soup.

Preparing as much as I can so the big things are done in advance is a huge help. For example, with a pot of rice already made and kale cleaned and chopped, all I have to do is sauté that kale and maybe make a side dish of tofu. Cooking in bulk can really make preparing dinner faster and easier. It also makes packing school or work lunches a lot easier, too.

ANSWERS FROM ERICA'S EXPERT

Culinary nutritionist Stefanie Sacks, MS, works hands-on with individuals and groups in transition to a healthier way of eating as a food counselor, nutrition educator, and chef instructor. She has been studying food and healing for twenty-five years, has her master's of science in nutrition from Columbia University, and is a graduate of the Natural Gourmet Institute for Health and Culinary Arts. Stefanie is noted for her unique expertise in creating a seamless translation of the most recent disease-specific medical science to a client's plate, with the kitchen as the centerpiece of education. Stefanie involves her clients in the day-to-day process of redefining their relationship with food to prevent illness and restore health. In Stefanie's private practice, she works intimately with clients in the comfort of their own homes. She also teaches and consults. She practices throughout the Hamptons, New York City, and the vicinity, and is the mother of two young children.

Nutrition

What does "natural" really mean when it comes to food?

The FDA claims to regulate the word *natural*. As per their regulations, it means foods that are:

- minimally processed
- free of any artificial ingredients including colors, flavors, sweeteners, or chemical preservatives
- in the case of meat and poultry, minimally processed using a method that does not fundamentally alter the raw products and free of artificial colors, flavors, sweeteners, preservatives, and ingredients that do not occur naturally in the food

But it's unclear what that last item really means, and the label should explain the use of the term *natural*. This is seemingly pretty straightforward, but it's actually very ambiguous, leaving it open to interpretation by food producers. It can basically mean whatever a company wants it to mean!

That said, as far as packaged foods are concerned, "natural" typically does hold true to its definition, but that doesn't mean there aren't "natural" flavors, colors, and high-fructose corn syrup in a food marked "natural." It doesn't mean that the food is devoid of genetically modified organisms (GMOs), which I'll explain in a minute. So pick and choose carefully. Also note that none of what I've just mentioned is too bad (except GMOs).

What is the definition of "organic"?
In a nutshell, according to the USDA, organic foods are those that are:

- produced using environmentally sound methods that don't utilize synthetic inputs such as pesticides
- devoid of GMOs
- not irradiated
- devoid of industrial solvents and chemical food additives including colors, flavors, sweeteners, and preservatives
- if livestock are involved, raised humanely with regular access to pasture and without the common use of antibiotics or growth hormones. In addition, their feed must be organic.

What are pesticides and why do we need to avoid them?
Pesticides, which include fungicides, herbicides, insecticides, and rodenticides, are chemicals used to kill harmful insects/animals or plants (such as weeds). Oddly enough, they are also harmful to humans. They are used primarily in agriculture and around areas where humans live—and thus are toxic to humans either from direct contact or as residue on food. They are also harmful to the environment because of their high toxicity. Pesticides are difficult to avoid unless you eat "100% organic" food (as defined here). Since this is not possible for most of the population, know that pesticides are okay to consume in small quantities. Do the best you can to avoid or minimize your exposure to them. (See my guidelines, in this question-and-answer section, on how to eat healthy without spending a lot of money.) Also make sure to wash fruits and vegetables thoroughly. For this, the good old-fashioned rule of thumb is

just fine: use water and your hands or a vegetable brush for scrubbing. When washing greens, fill a large bowl with water and place cut or whole greens in it for a soak, making sure to swish the vegetables around to remove the dirt. Pour the water out and repeat. When the water pours out clean, the greens are clean. (Sometimes you have to do this two or three times if the greens are really dirty, as with spinach.) Then either pat the leaves with a freshly cleaned dish towel or paper towel, or use a salad spinner to dry them.

What are preservatives, what is their purpose, and why do we need to avoid them?

The purpose of preservatives is to prevent spoilage, preserve the natural characteristics and appearance of food, and increase the shelf life of food for storage. As far as preservatives go, I break them into two categories: natural (good) and synthetic (bad). Some natural preservatives are salt, vinegar, sugar, and alcohol. The synthetic counterparts are benzoates (such as sodium benzoate and benzoic acid), nitrites (such as sodium nitrite), sulfites (such as sulfur dioxide), and sorbates (such as sodium sorbate and potassium sorbate). Natural preservatives *do not* need to be avoided, but synthetic ones do, for they are thought to be toxic to humans in some way, shape, or form—even though they are "generally recognized as safe" by the FDA. So take a careful look at your food labels! If not, you may never know what is lurking in your foods.

What are genetically modified foods, or GMOs (also called genetically engineered foods)?

GMOs are bacteria, plants, or animals whose DNA (genetic material) has been purposely altered, permitting selected genes to be transferred from one organism and into another—whether between related or nonrelated species. An example of a nonrelated gene transfer is when genes from shrimp, a cold-water species, are inserted into tomatoes to make those tomatoes resistant to frost. Bioengineering is used to create specific traits in crops that make them resistant to pests (for increased crop yield), to give a particular crop characteristics that are not inherent in their species (as in the tomato example), or to increase their nutritional value. The problem? We truly don't know the long-term effects of eating foods with altered DNA.

The four main GMO crops are:

- Corn
- Cotton
- Soybeans
- Wheat

Also (though not yet widely accepted by farmers but in existence):

- Beets
- Canola
- Papaya
- Potato
- Squash
- Sugar

These bioengineered foods are like tentacles taking over our food supply. Hundreds of millions of U.S. acres of farmland are devoted to growing genetically engineered foods. Although biotech companies proclaim GMOs safe for human consumption, I don't think we know enough about them to feel comfortable eating them.

What is irradiation?
Food gets "smashed" with irradiation to kill bacteria and molds that create spoilage so they look and taste fresh longer. Such foods can include fresh meat and poultry, which if irradiated is required to be labeled as such by the FDA. However, other foods that are irradiated don't have that requirement, such as wheat and wheat powder, white potatoes, many spices and dry vegetable seasonings, fresh eggs in the shell, and fresh produce. Although many people support the "merits" of irradiating food, food has been irradiated for years (about four decades), and irradiation is approved by the FDA, there are still many questions about irradiation that need to be answered, including: Are nutrients destroyed in the process? And do we experience any genetic damage from the possible by-products left in the food from the radiation?

Buying organic will confirm that food is not irradiated, and many dried herbs and spices that are not organic now note on their label that they are "nonirradiated."

What are processed foods and what are some suggestions for reducing the amount of processed foods consumed by my family?

By definition, foods that are altered in any way from their whole form—meaning everything from a sliced apple to packaged crackers—are processed foods. Whole foods, on the other hand, are those that are not altered in any way from their original state. You can reduce the amount of processed foods your family consumes by finding one day a week to cook a few things to keep in the fridge and freezer—such as soups and turkey meatballs. It's not an easy feat, but I make it happen even if it means putting my kids in front of the TV while I do it. Also, when buying foods, if the ingredient list is too long (five to eight ingredients or more) and if I can't pronounce an ingredient and/or don't know what it is, I don't buy it. Because I am so nitpicky about ingredients, I typically go for products with the fewest ingredients, thus ensuring they are the least processed. But I am no angel, so there are times when I do turn to more processed products; I just carefully select what those products are.

What is "healthy eating"?

I once had a client, Max, whose diet consisted of everything "bad" you can imagine, from daily red meat to processed "diet" foods. In contrast, another client, Meg, ate a diet rich in whole foods, with minimal amounts of processed foods, but had an "addiction" to diet soda and artificially sweetened gum. So, for Max, my goal was to minimize his red meat consumption to two to three times a week and replace 50 percent of his processed "diet" foods with healthier alternatives. For Meg, I focused on reducing her intake of diet soda and gum by slowly replacing both with more health-supportive options, such as seltzer with juice and gum sweetened with a sugar alcohol such as sorbitol (which is considered a natural sweetener, but if consumed in high amounts can cause digestive problems). My point is: "healthy" is a relative term and is different for everyone. However, in general, what I believe is central to the concept of healthy eating is to:

- Eat a diet of mostly whole foods. Again, whole foods are those foods that are not altered in any way from their original state.
- Include a variety of foods in your diet every day, meaning that your daily food intake should be comprised of whole grains such as rice or oats (or whole grain–based products), vegetables, fruits, protein such as legumes (beans), some animal products (if you choose), and healthy fats (such as olive or sesame oil).
- Eat breakfast, lunch, and dinner with snacks in between. Snacks can include but are not limited to fresh vegetables and fruits, nuts, seeds, cheese and crackers, soup, "healthy" cookies and milk, and whole grain chips with salsa.
- Try to avoid artificial ingredients (including sweeteners, preservatives, and flavors), dyes, and high-fructose corn syrup (HFCS). Though HFCS is considered "natural," it is highly processed and often comes from genetically modified corn.
- Buy organic if possible.
- Buy fish using the Monterey Bay Aquarium (www.montereybay aquarium.org) Seafood Watch as a guide—it's also available as a phone app—for the most updated information on the best seafood choices based on health and environmental impact.
- Buy local, even if not organic. Less travel to bring food to market means higher nutritional value. And you support local farmers.
- Buy lunch meats without nitrates or nitrites, chemical additives that preserve color and shelf life but are thought to be carcinogenic.
- Allow yourself to indulge once in a while! This means something different for everyone. For example, if you have a tendency toward eating junk foods (red meat, alcohol, cakes, cookies, and candy—you get the gist) then I suggest doing so once a week. (If not, you will rebel!) Otherwise, twice a month is fine. You have to determine this for yourself and base it on not only your relationship with food but also your overall health.

How can I eat healthy foods without spending a lot of money?

Eating healthily without spending a lot of money is all about negotiating. Here are a few suggestions:

- Seek out a "food cooperative," whether within the community, as with community-supported agriculture (CSA)—you pay a yearly membership fee and get a box of fresh local and many times organic vegetables weekly; an online cooperative; or an Internet grocery operation.

- If you're aiming for more organic choices, choose your fruits and vegetables with the Dirty Dozen in mind. This is the list of fruits and vegetables containing the most herbicide and pesticide residue. (Go to www.ewg.org for the most updated list; it's available as a phone app, too.) Also, frozen vegetables are not worse than fresh. So don't worry if you need to stock up on them. And if you can't go organic, don't beat yourself up. Eating conventional fruits and vegetables is better than not eating fruits and vegetables at all.

- If you're aiming for the healthiest animal foods outside of the obvious, most expensive organic option, go for those raised without hormones or antibiotics. Though these are fed a grain-based diet, they are typically treated more humanely.

- Buy fish that is local. Sometimes I buy frozen fish that often tastes just fine.

- Buying packaged foods that are organic is ideal but, again, not always possible. I always aim for those foods devoid of artificial ingredients (including sweeteners, preservatives, and flavors), dyes, and high-fructose corn syrup.

The bottom line: educated choices are the best choices!

Chapter 4

Getting Your Children to Eat Healthy

You can't say no to sugar all of the time, because that just makes kids want it really badly. I've learned to allow my children to have sugar only when they have something physical to do, and there's no chocolate in our house after 4:00 p.m., or they're up all night. Sugar is everywhere, so I am constantly reading ingredients. (Sometimes I feel more like the Sugar Police than a mom!) But I never give them sugar-free chemical stuff. I would rather they have the real thing than some chemical that has killed rats in labs. I have found many alternative products that don't do near as much damage and that my kids enjoy. I know there will always be ice cream at the mall. I just try to balance it all.

—Melissa Etheridge, mother of four

Recently, while my family was on vacation and I was driving Arianna and a girlfriend to the beach, I overheard the two girls talking in the backseat.

"Want to play a game?" Arianna asked her friend.

"Okay," her friend said. "What?"

"One of us picks a food, and the other person has to talk about it."

"Sugar," her friend suggested.

"It doesn't have any vitamins," said Arianna. "It breaks down your immune system. It's bad for your teeth."

I could barely contain my smile. Despite her occasional resistance to my teaching her about healthy food, Arianna had understood what I was saying. She'd heard me. That's all I can ask for. I have no answers as to how my kids will wind up eating later on in life, but as the hands-on parent that I am, I have to give them a healthy foundation. All I can do is introduce them to the right foods and take an active role in their well-being, so I can honestly say that I did my best and that I made an effort. That's all we can do as mothers, fathers, and caregivers.

But laying this healthy foundation wasn't easy. As I've mentioned, we did not start improving our way of eating until my son got sick. Before that, my children were typical American kids, eating what has become known as typical American fare: pizza, pasta, chicken fingers, mac 'n' cheese, and French fries. As picky eaters, they were used to canned soups, saltine crackers, chips, and gummy fruit snacks. Their only vegetables were broccoli with lemon, green peas, and overcooked collard greens at a soul food dinner a few times a year. They started the day with a glass of orange juice from a carton and cereals that I thought were healthy merely because they weren't sugar frosted. We enjoyed our desserts and had a Friday night ritual of ordering takeout pizza. (We still do, from time to time.)

But once Mina came into our lives, I had the challenge of changing my kids' palates. What made this more difficult was that I hadn't been raised on a macrobiotic diet. My mother did try to give us healthy food (for example, wheat bread instead of white), and she brought sweets into the house only once a month. (When she did, I thought it was because it was payday, but as an adult I realized that it was Mother Nature's monthly visit that had my mom craving sugar.) She also believed in cooking at home, because it was costly to dine out. But we certainly weren't eating tofu, miso soup, or kale.

But once I became a young adult, I loved my chocolate Frosty from the drive-through fast food restaurant and my apple pie from the place with the golden arches. I loved spilling my fast food French fries out onto the crinkly paper that came wrapped around my cheeseburger and smothering them in ketchup. I drank juice made from bright red powder, and orange soda, and ate those fried cheese puffs that turned my fingers bright orange. In college, candy bars, packaged cupcakes, and nacho chips were stashed in my backpack for my in-between class snacks. I did cook for myself, but not often. My point is that this new way of eating was an education for all of us—me included.

When it was time to change my kids' habits, I had to make a conscious decision that I was going to find the energy, push up my sleeves, and just do it. If I had thought about how hard it was going to be to change their meals from dinosaur-shaped chicken nuggets and pizza to kale, mushrooms, and whitefish, or if I'd thought about all the days ahead of me, I might have given up. I wasn't looking forward to turning our diets upside down, but I was looking forward to seeing the results. I knew it was not going to be simple. But I just kept telling myself that this was for our health.

My son, who was just three years old at the time, was my sugar child. He wanted sweets, such as candy and baked goods, and carbs, such as pasta, all the time. (And when I didn't know about his food sensitivities, I was loading him up on that stuff and pacifying him with the sweets he loved. I figured it was better for him to eat something rather than nothing.) So I thought he would be my challenge. I expected tantrums and withdrawal fits. I thought he'd fight me every step of the way. On the other hand, I thought my daughter was going to be easy. After all, she was older. But I had it all wrong. It was the total opposite. While my daughter resisted and fought me (and sometimes still does today), Addison took about two weeks to come around to our new way of eating. Even at the very young age of three, he recognized that when he ate better, he felt better. And that's when I realized that when it comes to food, the problem isn't the kids; it's the parents: We're the ones who say, "Oh no. They're not going to eat *that*." We psych ourselves into thinking that we have to give our children what they like or food that's "kid friendly" in order to get them to eat. We don't want the hassle. We don't have the energy for it, and so, without realizing it, we let our kids run the show.

I know this because these were the thoughts I had when Mina told me to kiss our familiar takeout pizza good-bye, go off animal protein, and start eating miso soup for breakfast! *She's out of her mind,* I thought. *How are my children going to go from eating pasta and chicken nuggets to miso soup and seaweed overnight?* (Mind you, my children had never had miso soup before or even heard of it.) But I was so desperate that I told myself to be open-minded and put my guard down.

During that year of our going macrobiotic, more Japanese products came into our home than I ever knew existed, and many of them are staples in my kitchen today. (See "Products Mentioned" for more information.) Many of these foods were foreign to my children. In fact, they probably knew less about Japanese food than many children their age, because my fish allergy had always kept us out of Japanese restaurants.

Before all this, the only beans they knew of were black beans, black-eyed peas, and pinto beans. Now I was buying adzuki beans (which are low in fat and sodium and high in protein, fiber, complex carbohydrates, iron, and potassium, and are believed to benefit the bladder, reproductive function, and kidneys; help prevent breast cancer; provide a good source of energy; promote regular bowel function; lower cholesterol; and tone the lungs). I also began buying sea vegetables such as arame, nori (typically used to make sushi rolls), agar, wakame, and kombu, which are full of fiber and important minerals naturally found in the ocean, such as iodine, magnesium, iron, phosphorus, potassium, and calcium. Instead of white rice, I bought short-grain brown rice—I was told it was easier for the body to digest—and instead of table salt, we used two things: one is called Sea Veg, which contains sea salt, kelp, and dulse, and the other is umeboshi vinegar, which is made from fermented plums. (Today my kids and I put umeboshi vinegar on a lot of our foods, such as kale, collard greens, and sushi. More on that in the recipes in "Really Easy Recipes Your Kids Will Love.") Daikon, a Japanese radish, also made it onto my regular shopping list. (Now daikon is like medicine to me, and something I try to keep in my home on a regular basis.) We also ate a lot of miso soup, because it's loaded with good bacteria. For that year, we stopped eating animal protein completely, and instead got our protein from sources such as tofu, tempeh, beans, and occasionally, our children would get freshwater fish such as grey sole and cod. Vegetable sushi also became a regular part of our diet. (And today my kids still love sushi.)

In addition to Japanese foods, we also started eating more roots and vegetables such as kale, parsnip, and rutabaga, which I'd never thought to purchase or serve my children.

If you are ready to change your children's diets, here are some of the guidelines I found helpful. My hope is that you'll find them helpful for you and your family, too.

Talk to Your Children About the Changes in Their Diets

I've always talked to my children as if they were adults, meaning no sugar-coating or using baby talk. So when it came to changing the way we were going to eat, I didn't ignore them or just use my authority and say, "We're eating this way because I'm the mom." It wasn't about power or control. It wasn't about being "the boss" or having to "win." It was about giving them nutrients through food and explaining this to them so they could understand, learn, and be more aware.

Then again, I didn't *ask* them to go along with me as we overhauled our diet. I told them, "This is what we're going to do." But I was very clear, honest, and as straightforward as I could be with a three- and a five-year-old. After all, this was going to affect their bodies and their taste buds, and I was respectful of that.

One thing that was very important to me was that my son and daughter not feel that this new way of eating was a punishment of some sort. For example, I didn't tell my son, "We're eating this way because of what you went through in the hospital." Instead, I told my kids that feeding them a healthy diet was part of my responsibility as their mother. "Mommy thought that what we were eating before was right for us and what I wanted to provide to you as a responsible mother," I explained. "But now I realize that some of those foods are not beneficial for us." Or I told them, "Mommy doesn't want you to be sad because you get sick and have to miss a birthday party or playdate. To prevent that, this is what we have to do." This wasn't one conversation, but several over time. As with many things in life, it was and still is a process. I reinforce our positive eating habits with these types of conversations even today.

I don't know what my children were thinking when I had these talks with them, but I do know that it was my responsibility to bring awareness to them and that you create this awareness by talking. I gave them concrete examples, such as saying to Arianna, "Do you notice how you get mucus after you eat ice cream, milk, or cheese? That's one of the side effects of dairy for you." One time, right after eating chicken nuggets at her former school, she got sick and had five days of diarrhea. I knew it was from the chicken nuggets, and I had to help her understand this. I explained the cause and effect between the chicken nuggets and her being sick. And she never touched the school's nuggets again! My kids will not eat everything that I put in front of them, but educating them has made them more open to eating nutrient-rich foods.

I explained which vitamins were in the foods they were eating and how those nutrients would impact their bodies. I had to find a way to engage them. For example, I'd tell Addison, "The calcium in this broccoli will make your muscles and bones strong." Sometimes when we eat a vegetable, we play a game. I ask them what nutrients they think are in that vegetable and what it does for our bodies. Then we look it up online together, so the kids can see if they're right, and they learn something about nutrition at the same time.

Eat with Your Kids Most of the Time

Even though the initial goal of this new way of eating was to improve my son's health, I decided to go along on the journey, too. I did this for a few reasons. First, I didn't want them to feel there was something wrong with them. Second, I'd have been a hypocrite if I'd told my children to eat one way while I ate another. (We tend to do this as moms, urging our kids to finish their broccoli and eat balanced meals while our "meals" consist of the leftovers on their plates, which we shove into our mouths while rushing to clean the kitchen, or the snack foods we pick on while making them dinner.) Last, I had my own health issues along with my allergies, so a healing diet could only help me, too. (And it did! My skin cleared up, I lost a few pounds, and my health conditions, such as a pain in my left arm, lumpy breasts, and ovarian cysts, improved.)

By day, I'm a busy mom, doing drop-offs and pickups, helping with homework, and taking my kids to playdates, after-school activities, and appointments. But once my children go to bed, my life changes. Because my husband's in the entertainment business, we often have last-minute dinners, fancy dress events, and charity functions to go to, and these are all places where food is served. Still, once we'd started our journey to wellness, I began eating dinner with my kids before an event. This not only improved my diet, but it helped my kids, because they actually saw that my eating habits were changing and that we really were in this together.

One note I should add here is about my husband. Though my son, daughter, and I went on this macrobiotic diet for a year, my husband did not. He tried it, but his lifestyle and work habits don't support the kind of strictness that our regime required. He works in shifts, and has frequent lunch and dinner meetings, so although he saw the benefits in the three of us and tried to go macrobiotic, it wasn't realistic for him to continue at that particular time.

Encourage Your Children to Try New Foods

Despite all the talking, my children didn't immediately agree to eat whatever appeared on their plates. Many times they said, "I'm not trying that," "What is this?" or "Ewww!" Other times they asked, "Why do we have to eat miso soup?" and "Do I have to eat that kale?" But even before going macrobiotic, I had a mantra when it came to food: "You get what you get and you don't get upset." My children had heard me say this so often that often one of them would say it to the other if he or she complained about a meal. "Our home is not a restaurant, and there's no chef here to take your orders," I also told them. There was one meal for the entire family and that was it. We all ate the same thing. (And still do.) If the kids gave me a hard time, I reminded them that the homeless man across the street would be happy to have the food they had in front of them. Whether they liked it or not, I said, we had to be thankful and appreciate what we were given. I kept this same mantra even when the food on our plates went from mac 'n' cheese and pizza to veggie sushi rolls and tempura. After all, I had to be the one to keep things positive, in perspective, and consistent. (As with many things in life, consistency is key.)

When my kids were trying the new foods, I'd encourage them to take one bite. If they didn't like it, I didn't force-feed them. And I never said, "You have to clean your plate." But I kept at it. Even if they didn't like a particular food the first time, I served it over and over again, hoping they'd like it in time. There are some foods that have been on our table a hundred times and they still won't touch them—such as green, leafy salads and tomatoes (despite the fact that they eat tomato-based products such as ketchup and tomato sauce). Other foods that have been on the table a hundred times, however, have gotten eaten and liked upon the umpteenth time, such as raspberries and blueberries.

I started small. I didn't serve my kids a big plate or a heaping pile of something new. This can be overwhelming, and wasteful if they don't like it. Instead, I'd serve a small portion. If they wanted more, I was happy to give it to them. And speaking of not wasting food, I always made sure that at least *I* liked the food they were trying, so in case they didn't like it, it wouldn't go to waste.

At times when I wanted my kids to retry a food they didn't like, I had to be creative. For example, one day I gave them baked butternut squash that was thinly sliced. They both tasted it, and neither of them liked it. The next night, I took the leftover butternut squash, warmed it in a pot, and then mashed it with a little bit of rice milk, maple syrup, agave, and cinnamon. And they ate it! I think that was because it was sweet and looked like mashed sweet potatoes, which they had had before.

There were times when I'd let a new food appear on my kids' plates without saying anything about it. I didn't make a big deal, because I didn't want to draw attention to it. Other times, when I saw the two of them exchanging looks—as in *What is this?*—I'd say, "I don't want to hear that you don't like the way it looks or don't want to eat it. Try it. Then if you don't like it, you don't have to eat it and you can talk about the taste."

I also tried to make my kids aware of their taste buds. Once, when I served Brussels sprouts, Addison turned to Arianna and said, "Do you think I'll like Brussels sprouts?" She had tried them and had not really cared for them. But before she could answer, I said to Addison, "Arianna's taste buds are different from yours. Let your taste buds tell you if they like Brussels sprouts or not." So he did. Though his taste buds told him they didn't like this new veggie, later that night he told my sister that "they weren't that bad." And Arianna, who had tasted the Brussels sprouts and said she really didn't like them, actually asked for some the next night. That's progress!

Let Your Kids Help with the Food Shopping

I started taking my children food shopping when they were young, so they would know where their food came from and could have contact with it. Each time they came to the store with me, I'd let them pick a new food. Something about their being able to choose something for themselves made it more interesting for them. This was how my daughter started eating raspberries. I told her it was time to try a new fruit. She chose raspberries, tried them, and liked them. (Unfortunately, on that same trip, my son picked kiwis and didn't like them.)

To make food shopping fun and educational, and keep my kids from getting restless, I'd relate it to reading and math. For example, I might say, "I need eight organic apples. Make sure they're Gala apples." They'd ask me how to spell *organic* and *Gala* and then started searching. They weren't wandering around the store by themselves, but this little bit of independence made them excited, and they felt as if they were helping. It was a team effort.

Make the fruit and vegetable section of the store the place where you let your kids help. The produce aisle is the nutrient-rich area. After all, in the snack aisle they're likely to be swayed by enticing pictures on the packages and grab junk food. I'd also prepare my kids by setting the tone before we entered the store: "We're going grocery shopping now. You get to pick some new fruits and vegetables and some cereal, and Mommy will do the rest of the shopping." This helped me get out of the store quickly.

Make Variations of Foods Your Kids Already Love

At one point my kids did not eat quinoa by itself. (Quinoa is a protein-rich grain that's great as a side dish or the base of a salad.) Then, one day, when they were eating the brown rice they loved and had been eating for a while, it hit me. I decided to try mixing quinoa with brown rice and see what

happened. I did, and they started eating it! Just the other night they ate quinoa by itself. I was so excited that I wanted to say something, but I also didn't
want to make too big a deal of it, so I stayed quiet (but inside I was smiling).
They now say, "Please pass the quinoa."

Bring Out the Condiments

Sometimes all it took to get my kids to try a new food was letting them experiment with condiments. For example, when it came to rice, sometimes we'd
put soy sauce on it. Or I'd let my son, who loves ketchup, put some on his
kale. If ketchup helped him get the vitamins from the kale, then it was fine
with me. I didn't do this every time he ate kale, but it's one way he used to
like it. Lemon was also a huge help. They loved squeezing a little juice from a
lemon wedge onto their vegetables.

    The point is it's about experimenting, finding ways to get kids to try new,
healthy foods without pouring sugar or salt on them. My kids know they're
eating broccoli or mushrooms, but sometimes there's a way they like to eat
that broccoli or those mushrooms, and that's fine with me. As long as they're
eating them, I'm not going to tell them how. That becomes a control thing.

Teach Them About Fruits and Veggies

A friend told me that her kids will not eat vegetables, so she juices their vegetables for them. Fresh vegetable juice is great, but it's also important to let
your kids see the veggies going into that juice. For example, my daughter
doesn't like blueberries and won't eat them on their own. But they're loaded
with antioxidants and other important nutrients, so I put them in her smoothies. She knows they're in there and she loves her smoothies, so it works. I do
this because I believe that when it comes to food, we need to expand our
children's horizons, because one day they're going to be making their own
food choices. If they don't see what they've been eating now, they may not
choose those fruits or vegetables when they're on their own, because it won't
be what they know. We tend to connect to things that are familiar to us. We

can teach them their fruits and vegetables the way we teach them their numbers, letters, and the four seasons. Don't we want our kids to be aware of different produce beyond the banana, orange, and apple they see at school or in picture books? Do we really want to limit them in this area?

Leave Room for Treats and Sweets

Do my kids get sweets and treats? Absolutely. I don't mind giving them dessert or a treat once in a while, but vitamins come before anything. If they want seconds of something at mealtime, the vegetable on their plates has to be gone first. For example, if we're having kale, brown rice, and turkey burgers, the kale better be gone before they ask for seconds of something else. I never say that they have to clean their plates or eat all their food; I don't believe in that. But they have to eat their vegetables.

I give occasional treats. For example, my kids love donuts from a New York City landmark that makes the only donuts my son can eat because of his allergies. So on a random Friday, I will go buy these huge, rich, gooey donuts as a treat for my kids. I don't mind my children having them occasionally, because I know what they had for breakfast that day and I know what they're going to have for dinner, which is likely loaded with nutrients. (And if it's not, that's okay, too. I don't beat myself up about it, because we don't eat donuts all the time.)

My daughter had her eighth birthday party at a well-known candy place in New York City. People were shocked that I, of all mothers, would let Arianna have her party there. When Arianna first asked me, I said no, because that place went against everything I believe in and who I am and all I want for my children. There aren't many nutrients in the entire place. The store offers tons of sugar, dyes, and chemicals, so why load my daughter or anyone else's kid up on that? But even after I said no, I kept thinking about it. I realized that I didn't want Arianna to grow up with the feeling that there was something lacking or to be made curious about a place by telling her it was off-limits. I decided to let her experience it now with little harm rather than let her curiosity about it possibly grow and become an issue later. That said, I did set some restrictions on how much candy and sugar the kids could have.

For example, I said okay to the candy goodie bags, but told the place that no soda or juice was to be served, and for dessert I had them serve only cake, no ice cream.

If I'm going to buy my kids or myself a treat that's a "packaged dessert," I look for the individually wrapped version. For example, instead of getting a full-size package of thirty cookies, we get the box that has individually wrapped portions. This gives us a limited, controlled amount to eat. When my kids get that package of cookies, they know exactly how many cookies they've got and that when they're done, that's it. And because the portions are wrapped, I can hide any extras in my pantry for another day. (These are the things we need to hide, not our kids' fruits and veggies.) The same applies to those rich, gooey donuts I mentioned: I bring home just one donut for each person in our family. We eat them, enjoy them, and move on. Limiting the amount really helps—as does baking your own sweet but healthy treats.

When we go to a restaurant or someone's house for dinner, I'm not a big stickler about what my children eat (except, of course, for the things they're allergic to). If they want mac 'n' cheese, a Shirley Temple, or dessert, I usually say okay. Why? Because I believe in balance. I know that 90 percent of what they're consuming is fresh, healthy, not processed, and mainly organic food.

I go for the real thing. If my kids want a treat, I don't pick the version that's fat-free or made with a sugar substitute. If we're going to do it, we do it old school. It may not be the healthiest, but often the ingredients that make a food fat-free or sugar-free are chemicals, which may be worse.

Don't Bring Home Unhealthy Foods

A mom I know asked me how I got my kids to eat healthy foods. "Sometimes I can't help but give my son those cookies we've got," she said in a frustrated tone of voice. But if you bring unhealthy food into the home or have a cabinet filled with junk food, then that's what your kids are going to want. If you don't have those things in the house or have a limited selection, then there's not much to argue about. We're doing more of a disservice to our kids by having junk in the house.

Find Teachable Moments

One day, when Arianna was getting ready for school, she said, "Mom, if you could eat only dairy for the rest of your life or eat only carbs for the rest of your life, which one would you pick?" I didn't respond with "I don't know why you're asking me this. I don't eat that stuff and don't know why you eat it." I realized it was a moment to shed some light and bring awareness to her. And I took advantage of it. "Well, let's see. Dairy may cause inflammation, tumors, mucus, and skin rashes," I said, loving that moment. "But carbs can make me gain weight, swell up, and get constipated. You know what? They're both not great, but I think I'll go for the carbs." I wanted to explain the difference between the two, but I didn't want her to feel that I was lecturing her. In that answer, I felt I was teaching her something.

Teach Your Kids to be Thankful for Their Food

In my house, we always thank God for the food that's before us. My kids are aware that they're about to enjoy a meal, but that there are people somewhere else in the world who are going hungry. I try to bring the awareness to them that there's a child in the world who has nothing. Before each meal, we also say, "Thank you, God, for today. Thank you, God, for this food. Amen." We thank God no matter where we are or whom we're with. We say our prayer in hotels and restaurants, too.

I've taught my children never to say, "I'm starving." If they do, I'll ask, "Did you eat today? Did you eat yesterday?" They will nod yes. Then I'll explain: "So you're not starving. There are people who don't have what you had yesterday or today." I remember my daughter, when she was about seven years old, saying, "Mommy, I almost told you I'm starving. But instead I'm going to tell you that I'm very, very hungry." I had to smile, because she'd gotten it.

Choose Your Words Carefully

I try not to say "bad" when it comes to food, or "bad for you." I also make a conscious effort never to say things such as "If you eat that, you're going to get fat" or "That food will keep you skinny." I don't discuss weight, and I make sure to explain that the way I use the word *diet* in our home means "a way of eating," not a way to lose or gain weight. Weight does not matter; being healthy does. I try to link food to my children's health in a positive way and tell them what vitamins they're getting from it.

Don't Use Food for Emotional Reasons

I can't be responsible for how my children choose to soothe themselves or celebrate later in their lives, but as their mother and primary caregiver it is my job to introduce them and expose them to certain things in life. So I try not to link food to emotions. For example, I never say, "Your feelings got hurt, let's go for ice cream" or "You're home sick from school, so let's make cupcakes." On the flip side, I also don't say, "You did well on that test, let's get a donut" or "You were so good at your competition, here's a lollipop." Food isn't a Band-Aid. I don't use it as any kind of reward or as a way to discipline. (The fact that teachers reward with candy is something I have a big issue with.) If my children feel sad, I tell them to write about it, draw about it, or get their emotions out in another way. *Go scream or hit your pillow. Go find something to do to release it.* If it's time to celebrate or reward them, I do it with free hugs and kisses, a card with a positive uplifting message, or a little trinket. My goal is to use food in its simplest form and for the reason it was produced: that is, to nourish the mind, body, and soul, and I'm clear about sharing this with them. I often say, "We eat because it's what our bodies need for fuel. We eat to keep moving and grooving." Reminding kids that what they put in their bodies impacts how they feel is important. But how will they know this if we don't tell them?

Strive for Balance

I make an effort not to deprive my children in any way, and I don't force them to eat anything they don't enjoy once they've tried it. You have to find an eating plan that works for you and your child. The healthy way will become a way of life for you and your family if you just keep at it. I'm not extreme. I try to find balance. Sometimes it's hard, and it doesn't happen every day. But living a healthy life *is* possible. And an attempt is better than no attempt.

None of this was easy, but it has all been worth it. After all, our pediatrician went from seeing my kids, especially Addison, several times a month to seeing them once a year for their school physical. Initially, the pediatrician was surprised by this and actually asked me if I had been seeing another doctor. I just smiled at this sign of how far we had come and assured her that the only major change we had made was in our diet. Now when she sees us for those annual visits, she tells my children, "That diet your mom has you on must be working." And I agree with her. The changes took work, but they have made a big, I mean a *huge*, difference in my children's physical health and their behavior—and in my own.

ANSWERS FROM ERICA'S EXPERT

Fred Pescatore, MD, is a traditionally trained physician who practices nutritional medicine and is the author of several well-known books on the subject, such as *The Allergy and Asthma Cure*, *Feed Your Kids Well*, *Boost Your Health with Bacteria*, and the *New York Times* bestseller *The Hamptons Diet*. Pescatore is president of the International and American Association of Clinical Nutritionists and head of Medicine 369, an integrative medical facility in New York City.

Kid-Friendly Eating Tips

What if your child is a picky eater?

Food is one way our kids test us the most. We don't allow them not to brush their teeth or take a bath. But when it comes to food, they push us as far as they can—and we let them get away with it. Research shows that you have to introduce a food twenty-five times (and have them taste it twenty-five times) before children will take to it, because they need to get used to it. Unfortunately, this is where many parents give up. But I promise you that if you put a food on the table often enough, they'll eventually eat it and even begin to like it. (This conclusion comes from many years of experience working with parents and their children.) One thing you can do is if your child likes a food such as spinach but doesn't like or won't try kale, you can mix the two together. Start with 90 percent spinach and 10 percent kale. The next time, make it 80 percent spinach and 20 percent kale; then 70 percent spinach and 30 percent kale; and so on, until they're eating mostly kale.

It's important that you're adamant about your children sticking to a healthy diet. You have to be firm. Rest assured, your child is not going to starve. You're not a bad parent when you say, "You either eat this or you don't eat" or "You have to finish your greens." You're actually a better parent. There are also some fun ways you can work with healthy food. Try cauliflower mashed potatoes or make chicken fingers using brown rice flour and then bake them. They're really good. Also, the earlier you start giving them healthy food, the better off you are, because they will develop a taste for it. Things such as kale, brown rice, and tofu will taste normal to them. Also, variety is an important part of everyone's diet, but especially for our kids. They are learning so much about the world every day. It's up to us to broaden and enrich their lives as much as we can.

What are the worst foods and drinks you can give kids?

Unfortunately there are many, but the worst offenders are:

- **Soda.** Not only is it a chemical, but it also makes your child's bones brittler. And diet soda is no better than regular soda. Aspartame has been linked to hundreds of brain development issues in children, and Splenda has been linked to brain deficits. Why give your children anything to stop their brain development? If your child wants a drink that gives her a fizzy feeling, try flavored seltzer.

- **Sugar.** Sugar can cause many adult health problems with roots that begin in childhood. This sweetener suppresses the immune system, causes tooth decay, and can lead to behavioral issues, hormonal imbalances, and obesity, among other problems. Plus, sugar is nutritionally barren. In most cases, the sugar we eat satisfies our hunger, thereby leaving no room for foods with real nutritional value. It's just not healthy. Unfortunately, the average elementary school kid eats 33 teaspoons of sugar a day, and the average teenage boy eats more than 149 pounds of sugar a year! This seems hard to imagine, but much of this sugar is consumed in disguised forms. It isn't just in candy; it's hiding in foods such as fruit juice, milk, cereal, preservative-packed snacks, bread, baked beans, ketchup, pastas, and pasta sauce. It's easy to see how it adds up. There are many other words for sugar to look for on ingredient lists. For instance, *honey, concentrated fruit juice, barley malt, maple syrup, agave, rice syrup, cane sugar,* and *fructose.* Take a look at food labels and if you see anything that ends in *-ose* or *-ol,* that's sugar, too.

- **Wheat.** If we didn't eat wheat we'd all be about 80 percent healthier. Wheat is a processed food, and by processing it you're getting rid of all the nutrients, especially the grain itself. As a result, it's high in calories but low in nutrients. Also, a lot of people have food sensitivities or allergies to wheat and don't even realize it. I suggest eating alternative grains such as buckwheat, amaranth, quinoa, spelt, and kasha.

- **Fruit juice.** It's loaded with sugar, offers no nutrients, and study after study after study has shown that the more fruit juice kids drink, the fatter they are and the more likely they are to be diabetic. Many well-meaning parents have leaped to the mistaken conclusion that substituting fruit juices for soda is healthier. But this is a dangerous misconception. After all, sugar behaves in the body the same way no matter how it's delivered. As far as I'm concerned, there is absolutely no nutritional value in fruit juice. The vitamin C you can get from a glass of juice is too small an amount to compensate for all the sugar that juice contains.

Why is fast food so harmful for kids?

It sets kids up to be unhealthy because there's nothing good about it. It contains a lot of fat and sodium and has no nutritional value. The meat has growth hormones in it, which can cause obesity and possibly cancer, and the potatoes are planted in soil that has no nutrients. Not to mention that the acrylamide that's formed during the frying is known to cause cancer. Nobody should have French fries or pizza every day. It should be an occasional treat, and as soon as you get your kids (and yourself) out of the fast food habit the better. Plus, you can make healthy versions of fast food, such as chicken fingers, at home. (See the recipe for Chicken Strips on page 199.)

Why are processed foods considered unhealthy?

During processing, natural vitamins and minerals are taken out of the food. At best, they are replaced with chemical versions that the body cannot readily or completely absorb and thus are nutritionally useless. At worst, these natural nutrients are not replaced at all. The aim of food manufacturers is to produce food more cheaply and with a longer shelf life, but the result is food that is not as healthy for us as it was in its original state. In many respects, food processing has made it possible to feed more people than ever before. Unfortunately, processed foods are often prepared with partially hydrogenated vegetable oil, which has been proven to lead to an increased number of health risks, such as heart disease, high cholesterol, and obesity.

What do you tell adults who say, "Oh, they're just kids. They're young, so what they eat now doesn't matter"?

Nothing could be further from the truth. Actually, what your children eat now is vital to what they're going to eat later. That's the key. This is the time when their bodies are forming, and food is the most critical part of that. If their bodies don't form correctly now, they're only going to be in trouble later. More often than not, people don't outgrow the eating patterns they set as children—they will have them for the rest of their lives. As parents, we are generally aware that the habits, values, and disciplines we instill in our children will serve them throughout their lives. Yet oddly enough we cling to the misguided notion that in terms of their eating habits, children are a species apart from the rest of the human race that commonsense rules and well-established laws of cause and effect do not apply. Eating is just habits. So if you learn good habits as a child, they'll stick with you for a lifetime. It takes dedication and hard work to instill proper eating habits in children. But in the end they will appreciate it, and so will you. That said, it's also never too late to introduce healthy eating.

My child loves and craves sugar. How can I help him kick this habit?

Slowly start weaning him off it, because you can't expect a child to quit cold turkey when he's used to sweet treats. For example, give him ten M&M's today, nine M&M's tomorrow, eight the next day, and so on. Then make sugar a treat, not an everyday food.

Why don't you believe in cow's milk for kids?

Cow's milk is just awful. It undergoes the processes of pasteurization, which may destroy any of its nutritional value, and homogenization, which makes the fat and cholesterol present in the milk more susceptible to oxidation and the formation of free radicals. (Free radicals have been associated with tumors, autoimmune and other destructive diseases, and many body-damaging processes.) Cow's milk swells us up and leads to more mucus in our system, and it has thirteen grams of sugar in a serving. Cow's milk is also extremely allergenic, probably the number one allergen for most children. Although milk is touted as a great source of calcium, something a growing child needs, you can get much more calcium in dark, green leafy veggies such as kale, Swiss chard, and broccoli, and from peanuts and fish skin. Also, milk, along with foods such as eggs that are not organic, can contain growth hormones, which may be one reason one-third of our children are obese, why girls are menstruating at the age of seven, and why some boys are growing breasts.

But you have alternatives. You can give your kids unsweetened soy or rice milk or even almond milk. These are much less allergenic than cow's milk. If you start to give your kids these drinks early enough, they'll never know the other thing exists. But if they've had regular milk for a while now, then don't switch immediately from cow's milk to soy milk. It will taste different, and your child will know the package is different from what he's used to. Instead, do what I mentioned with the spinach and kale: start with 80 percent cow's milk and 20 percent almond or soy milk. Then go to 70 percent cow's milk and 30 percent almond or soy milk, and so on.

Why is it so important to eat seasonal foods?

There are several reasons:

- When you eat foods that are not in season, they often travel from far, far away to get to you. If you just start with the obvious, it's ruining the environment to have all this food come from five thousand miles away.
- Plus, we don't have any control over the pesticides and herbicides that are used in other countries. In fact, many of the chemicals used in other countries are banned in the United States.
- Often the foods that come from far away have to be picked earlier and aren't ripe when picked, so chemicals are used to preserve them.
- When these foods have to travel a long way to get to us, they can lose nutrients.
- The other important part of eating with the seasons is that I believe that we are part of our environment, and our bodies are attuned to doing different things during different seasons. If you think back to when we were cavemen, that's what we did. That's what made hunters and gatherers so healthy. They didn't have a 747 plane flying pineapple in from Hawaii in the winter. No. They ate what was right for those months and what was available. Genetically, we're not that far from cavemen. I don't think that our bodies are made to digest pineapple and mango in the middle of winter in New York City.

What are some tools I can use to help my child change his eating habits?

Before I see a patient, I have him or the parents keep a food diary, which is a record of everything he's eaten for anywhere from three days to a week. This includes snacks (even gum), meals, and beverages. Before your child embarks on a new nutritional lifestyle plan, keep a food diary. Then go over the changes you'll make in this old routine. Circle trouble spots or those items that will change when you alter his diet, and mention foods or drinks that are healthy replacements for these circled items. This way your child will know that he has control over what he's eating and it will encourage his active participation. You can also talk to your child about potential healthy eating obstacles and make a list of healthy foods your child can eat. (You can even have a contest to see who can add more foods to this list.) Doing all this makes your child part of the solution, rather than part of the problem, which boosts your chances for success.

How do you avoid the colds and flus that go around school each year?

Eat right! Eating wrong is why kids are sick all the time. Take sugar and yeast out of your kid's diet—these ingredients suppress the immune system. (When *Candida albicans*, a naturally occurring yeast in the body, is allowed to overgrow, I believe it can be detrimental to the health of many people, including children.) Yeast is found in breads, except those that say they're "yeast-free," but if you want a yeast-free diet, you also need to eliminate sugars and high-carbohydrate vegetables such as potatoes, peas, corn, and lima beans. Also, give your children a good probiotic: good bacteria that keep the stomach really healthy. (A child can be given a probiotic as young as three months old. Start with a powder.) This is important, because that's where 80 percent of your immune system forms. Eat real, whole foods as much as possible. Eat if it grows out of the ground or swims in the ocean, but if man has touched it, run far away from it! This is what I tell the kids I see in my practice—and they're never sick, they never catch colds, and they're never out of school.

Why is it important to give your child a probiotic whenever they take an antibiotic?

Probiotics are really the opposite of antibiotics. They're good, healthy, useful bacteria that unfortunately get removed along with the harmful bacteria whenever your child takes an antibiotic. It is necessary for the human intestine to maintain a critical balance among all the different bacteria present in the digestive system. Whenever one becomes unbalanced, symptoms may occur. After all, these bacteria play a vital role in supporting and protecting intestinal and immune function. The three most common protective strains of bacteria are *Lactobacillus acidophilus*, *Bifidobacterium bifidum*, and *Lactobacillus bulgaricus*. I usually prescribe a product that contains all three.

What's the best beverage for my kids to drink?

Water is the gold standard for drinking. And I encourage you to make this your children's sole beverage (and your own). A good habit for your child to get into is to drink fluids constantly during the day. Even if you don't feel thirsty, it's still important to drink water. Water is essential to life. It helps regulate body temperature, cushion joints, remove toxins, maintain strength and endurance, protect organs and tissues, and carry nutrients to every cell in the body. By the time you are actually thirsty, you are already mildly dehydrated. Some common symptoms of chronic dehydration are headache, fatigue, flushed skin, light-headedness, and dry mouth. It is believed that during chronic dehydration, the body produces more histamine, substances that contribute to many allergic reactions. My rule of thumb is that a person should drink in ounces of water their body weight in kilograms. One kilogram equals 2.2 pounds, so to get your child's weight in kilograms, just divide the weight by 2.2. For example, if your child weighs 88 pounds, this is 40 kilograms, so he or she should be drinking at least 40 ounces of water a day. This total does not include any other beverage, except herbal decaffeinated tea and club soda.

What are other tips for setting good eating habits?

- Never force your child to finish everything on his plate. This just sets up a bad eating pattern. The pressure to eat everything on your plate, day after day, will only encourage a pattern of overeating or, worse yet, another type of eating disorder.
- Food is food, and that's all it is. Don't give it any other connotation. We constantly have to be aware of whether we are using it as a reward or punishment. In the long run, food bribery creates far more problems than it solves.
- Buy only the foods you want your child to eat and allow him to make his own choices from this selection.

or smiling back at me, I saw blood. A lot of it. The blood was all over her face, nightgown, and crib. It covered the sheet and bumpers. At first I didn't know where it came from, but once I'd cleaned her up I realized it was coming from her chin. I thought this was just a onetime incident, but to my surprise it happened the next morning, too. And the next. This continued for months. (The amount of blood was so unbelievable that I actually took pictures of it to show the pediatrician and other doctors we consulted.) I took her to our pediatrician and several dermatologists, who told me that Arianna had contact dermatitis. This is when the skin gets inflamed after it comes in direct contact with an irritating substance. Arianna's skin had obviously gotten so itchy and uncomfortable that she had been scratching her chin while she slept, and all that scratching had caused her chin to bleed. The dermatologists we saw prescribed various creams, but none of them worked, not even a topical steroid. So Arianna continued to scratch her chin on and off for another year and a half.

I became convinced that the cause of this irritation was something she was being exposed to at home, so I became like a detective trying to determine what that "something" was. Since her chin was always bloody after a night's sleep, I figured that something in her room must be bothering her. This reminded me of a skin irritation I experienced right after I graduated from college. At this time in my life, I was trying to figure out what to do with my future. Having recently moved out of my college apartment, a girlfriend let me stay with her while I figured out my next steps. Within a short period after arriving at her house, my skin started breaking out and itching like crazy. I remember sitting next to her on the sofa watching TV while constantly scratching myself like an animal with fleas. This went on for weeks. Then one day I asked my friend if she'd mind if I cleaned her apartment while she was at work. (Her apartment looked good aesthetically, but I knew it needed to be cleaned.) Once she said yes, I rolled up my sleeves and vacuumed, dusted, and scrubbed that place from top to bottom. I wiped on top of the fridge and mopped under the furniture. While I cleaned, I noticed that every room had one of those plug-in air fresheners, the kind that contain a hardened, jellylike substance and have a strong, perfumed odor. I had a lightbulb moment that this was the problem, so I unplugged one of them, took a whiff, and—it had a strong perfume odor that stung my nose. With my friend's permission, I unplugged and tossed out all the air fresheners. I also changed the laundry detergent I was using, buying one that was free of fragrance. Within a few days, I noticed subtle changes. And over time, the itching subsided and my skin was back to normal.

But that wasn't my only experience with skin problems. Starting in college and for several years after graduating, I lived with a horrible rash under both my armpits. It came and went for four years, and although I moved from Colorado to Atlanta to California during that time, not one dermatologist whom I consulted helped. Each doctor gave me a topical cream that worked for a couple of days—maybe two to three weeks, tops—but then the rash always returned during warm weather. Clearly, this temporary fix wasn't addressing the root of the problem. I found myself becoming dependent on a cream, and whenever the weather got hot, the rash got worse. Even with this rash, I told myself that I still had to shave under my arms, because I was not going to have an ugly rash *and* hairy armpits.

Still, my armpits were so smelly and horrible looking, really an embarrassment, and my skin itched so much that I'd wake up with blood under my fingernails from all the scratching I was doing while sleeping. On top of all this, the pain of that raw, irritated skin was unbearable. I wanted to cry because I was so uncomfortable. (Thank God I didn't have a man in my life at the time, because that rash would have sent him running!) When I moved to Southern California, where the climate calls for tank tops, sundresses, and bathing suits, I didn't know what to do.

Finally, my cousin, who worked in television production, told me about someone named Majid Ali, a licensed acupuncturist and Chinese herbalist whom her coworker had raved about. (Though he's not a doctor, I personally refer to him as Dr. Majid.) I was skeptical. But because past dermatologist visits, a biopsy, and a trip to the emergency room hadn't helped, I figured I had nothing to lose.

As it turns out, I had a lot to gain. Dr. Majid was the first person who exposed me to anything besides Western medicine, and at that time I hadn't met anyone as in tune with and aware of the human body as he was. He asked me if I shaved my armpits, and I said yes. Then he asked me if I left my razor in the shower when I was not using it, and if I shared the shower with a roommate. The answer to both those questions was yes. He explained that leaving the razor in the shower left it susceptible to germs, which had the potential to cause irritation. He also explained that shaving my armpits opened my skin up and therefore allowed the toxic ingredients from my deodorant (such as the heavy-metal aluminum) and those germs to enter my body. Now my body was trying to release those toxins where they were being applied.

Dr. Majid also told me something I had never heard before. He said, "You need to change your diet and detox." *Hmm, what does that mean?* I wondered. He suggested herbs that were disgusting in taste but that turned out to be a miracle and a blessing. I had to put a scoop of these ground-up herbs in my mouth and then flush them with water. He also advised me to avoid all dairy and yeast and to increase my plain water intake profusely. I also had to eat spelt instead of wheat, and give up the acidic orange juice I had been drinking every morning in favor of a specific brand of organic apple juice (R.W. Knudsen). "Everything you're eating is feeding your condition," he told me.

Yes, the herbs were disgusting, and I knew it would be hard to give up foods I ate daily, but I was so desperate for a solution. No other doctor had mentioned anything that Dr. Majid had. Still, he warned me, "Things will become worse before they get better, because the toxins need to be released." Well, he was right. The rash spread all the way down to my wrists, turned a purplish-blue color, and had a sour smell to it. At first I was angry at Dr. Majid, frustrated that once again there was no solution. *Maybe he doesn't know what he's talking about,* I thought.

But I didn't give up, and within a month or so of detoxing, and with this new way of eating, the rash slowly started to dissipate. Eventually it was 100 percent gone, and for good. I was thrilled. Actually, I was *shocked*. Four years of living with this, using creams that didn't always work, dealing with burning, bleeding, constant scratching, and a foul odor, and finally it was all over. I haven't picked a razor up since then—I only wax my armpits now—and I don't use any deodorant; only rose water when needed. Looking back, I see that Dr. Majid not only helped me in the short term with my armpits, but he also prepared me for the long term, because he opened my eyes to alternatives to Western medicine, made me aware of the impact of toxins in our bodies, and made me understand how simple changes with foods can make a lifelong difference.

These two past personal experiences convinced me that Arianna's chin irritation was most likely a result of some sort of toxin or irritant trying to escape her body. And so I got to work making changes in our home to help eliminate those toxins. I started by looking at where she spent her time, viewing everything as a potential culprit. It became a guessing game.

Arianna was my first child and a baby girl, so I had gone all out when I decorated her room. She had thick, pale-pink plush carpeting and long, heavy, fancy drapery. She had an overstuffed chair with pretty pillows and adorable, plush stuffed animals perched on her shelves and floor. But once her skin irritation began, I had to opt for a healthy child over a pretty little girl's room. So I made changes, lots of them. At first I felt a little kooky doing all these things and turning the house upside down to figure out what was bothering my daughter, but it was worth it. I believe these changes are what stopped her skin irritation, and I think it probably made us all healthier, too. What follows are the steps I took to do what I called "de-junking my home." My home is now completely de-junked.

Start with the Bed

MATTRESS AND PILLOWS

The mattress was one of the closest things to Arianna's face while she slept. So I encased it in a dust mite cover. Dust mites are microscopic organisms that are believed to be one of the most common triggers of allergy symptoms such as itching, sneezing, sniffling, congestion, and inflamed or infected skin; they're also believed to make asthma worse. In order to grow and reproduce, dust mites feed off the dead skin cells our bodies naturally shed, and they need moisture. Since we spend long stretches of time in our beds, shedding skin cells and sweating and breathing while we sleep, our pillows, mattresses, and bedding make ideal homes for dust mites. Though there's no way to get rid of them in pillows and mattresses for good, an allergy cover at least put a barrier between Arianna and these microscopic critters, because the covers are woven in such a way that even dust mites can't slip through.

When Arianna got older and started sleeping with a pillow, I bought hypoallergenic pillows and encased them in dust mite covers, too.

BEDCLOTHES

I traded traditional baby laundry detergent for a natural product made without chemicals. While I was pregnant, I was like most moms who stocked up on the baby detergent recommended for newborns. I loved it because it smelled sweet and fresh, and like many of us, I had been conditioned to think that "fresh" baby scent meant that my clothes, sheets, towels—and my baby—were clean. (Looking back, I find that so silly, because babies naturally smell clean, fresh, and pure on their own. They don't need any extra scent enhancement.) But those smells are actually chemicals and fragrances, which can be irritating for some people. The tricky part is that you may not know you are bothered by these things, because the discomfort can be so subtle (for example, a headache, burning eyes, tingling in the throat, sniffling, sneezing, coughing). Fabric softeners also contain those ingredients, so I stopped using them as well. Instead, I used a natural product that was chemical- and fragrance-free. (Note: Make sure the product says "unscented," not "fragrance free." "Fragrance free" actually means the manufacturer has used a chemical ingredient to mask the product's scent, and that masking agent can be irritating, too.)

At least once a week, I washed my daughter's sheets and dust mite covers in hot water—as opposed to warm—because hot water helps kill dust mites. I also put them in the dryer on high heat.

Look at the Walls

Arianna's walls were a beautiful shade of pale rose pink with a colorful mural of angels painted on them. (Because she's my angel.) But I had no idea if the painters had used nontoxic paint, and if they hadn't, perhaps something Arianna was breathing in was irritating her. So I had her room repainted with a water-based paint, which is more environmentally friendly. It was a hassle and a big inconvenience, but her health was the priority.

Get Rid of the Dust

CARPETING

Arianna's room had a thick pink carpet that she sat on all the time. It was beautiful and very girly, but during my search to find out what was bothering her skin, I learned that carpeting is actually one of the worst things to put in a child's room. The fibers can hold on to potential allergens such as dust, mold, dust mites, and dirt. Sometimes you can't get rid of these things just by vacuuming. In fact, vacuuming can bring them to the surface of a carpet and send them into the air.

I took baby steps here. First, I got rid of the plush, wall-to-wall carpeting and went with an area rug—an adorable rug with Spanish on it so Arianna could learn the words. I loved it. But when the rash did not go away, I got rid of the area rug and went to bare wood floors. They're not as comfortable to sit on, but they didn't pose the same risk as her sitting on carpeting with hidden dust—or so I thought. A few years later, I realized that our hardwood floors had had polyurethane applied to the surface. This chemical is believed to give off compounds that may cause lung irritation, among other health issues. By now Addison had been born and was sharing the room with Arianna, so I found an eco-friendly website and ordered individual bamboo tiles to cover the wooden floors. (They weren't as cute as my Spanish rug, but they are healthier.)

CURTAINS AND DRAPES

Arianna's long, pretty drapes had to go, too, since they were also a place for dust to collect. They were made of thick, heavy, floor-length fabric that couldn't go in the washing machine, so therefore they did not get washed regularly. All I could do was pat them clean, and they still released little puffs of dust when I did so. Instead, I got blackout shades and sun shades, which are easy to wipe down and don't hold dust the way drapes do.

STUFFED FRIENDS

One of the hardest parts of this detox was getting rid of all Arianna's stuffed animals. They were cute, adorable, and exactly what you'd imagine in a sweet little girl's room. She didn't sleep with them, but they rested in her crib during the day. One that I really loved was an oversize pink stuffed dog from the well-known toy store FAO Schwarz, which sat in the corner of her room. It was so big and comfortable that one day Arianna took a nap on it. Unfortunately these adorable animals can harbor dust mites, dust, and other things that can make you sneeze, wheeze, itch, and break out in a rash. Even though we took them out whenever she slept in her crib, there was still a chance that they'd leave allergens behind, and that was a chance I didn't want to take.

Today, my kids do own a few stuffed animals, but I don't allow them in their beds. I tell them, "It's very cute, but this furry thing has dirt in it that we can't see. We don't take dirty things to bed." If your child does have an animal he can't part with, make sure to machine-wash it regularly in hot water and use high heat in the dryer to help kill any possible dust mites. You can also put stuffed items that aren't machine-washable—such as animals and decorative pillows—in the freezer for a couple of hours at a time. Yes, the freezer: the extreme cold helps kill dust mites.

BLANKETS

Even though Arianna was just a baby and didn't sleep with any blankets, she received several beautiful ones as gifts. They were made of all sorts of fabrics, and some were even personalized with her name or initials. I used a few of the personalized ones in her stroller when I took her for a walk, because they did not have direct contact with her skin; I'd put them on top of the clothing she was wearing. I stored the rest of them as keepsakes and donated the others.

Turn Your Home into a "No Shoes" Zone

Anyone who came to our house took his or her shoes off before walking in the door. (This rule still applies.) Whether you live in New York City or out in the country, your shoes can track chemicals such as asbestos, rodent repellent, dirt, dog poo and pee, and allergens onto the floor where your children play, crawl, and drop toys before putting them in their mouths. (If you have pets, they probably lick the floors, too.)

Along those lines, I also don't let anyone sit on our beds with clothes worn outside (which we call "outside clothes"). Just like your shoes, your clothes can carry dirt from outside, bedbugs, and things such as pollen, which can trigger allergies. We never sit on the bed with outside clothes, but there are times when my husband will come home and lie on the bed. That is, until my kids say, "Daddy get up. You have outside clothes on!"

Look at Your Cleaning Products

READ THE LABEL

The next step in my de-junking was to look under my kitchen sink and start reading the labels of the products I had been using. Most of them were filled with chemicals, which can then get on my plates, drinking glasses, skin, furniture, and the bathtub. For example, when I used to use that dishwasher rinse that helps prevent spots on glasses, it left a residue I didn't always see with my naked eye. I noticed this when I saw the residue coming off when I'd put the glass underwater. So when I realized there was a chance that my daughter and, later, my son were at risk for ingesting these chemicals or having them touch their skin, I stopped using the rinse, or traditional dishwashing liquid and powder, and opted for eco-friendly brands such as Seventh Generation.

USE NATURAL PRODUCTS

In addition to eco-friendly dishwashing products, I started cleaning my house with a mixture of water and vinegar, which I poured into spray bottles. I used this (and still do) for the floors and windows. It's not the best-smelling thing, but it works without chemicals. I also used Dr. Bronner's Pure Castile Liquid Soap, in peppermint, to mop the floors, clean out the refrigerator, wash the tub, and wipe down the countertops. It is chemical-free, so you can even bathe with it.

I would also rinse the tub quickly before letting my kids climb in for baths. I didn't want them soaking in the residue from the cleaning products used there. This isn't going to cause any major problems, but with a child who has sensitive skin, it could be an irritant, and I didn't want to take the chance.

I also got rid of bleach. I know it's believed to be a good way to clean, especially those household germs. But I didn't want that strong, dangerous chemical in my home, and I certainly didn't want to use it to clean the toys that Arianna and Addison were most likely going to put in their mouths.

To clean those items, once a week I'd fill the bathtub with hot water and a chemical-free detergent (such as Seventh Generation or Dr. Bronner's) and soak their toys. Sometimes I'd add vinegar or baking soda to the water. (Arianna loved doing this with me. It was fun for her to throw all her toys in the tub.) Then we'd let the toys soak overnight, give them a good rinse in the morning, and set them out to air-dry on a towel. I also got rid of the plastic squeeze toys (such as rubber duckies) that trap water inside them. I did this after I noticed dark areas inside the toys where you could see through the plastic. That was where mold was growing because the toy was a closed environment with moisture in it.

I stopped using carpet cleaners and powders that contained chemicals. These can be potentially harmful to children. (More on this in the "Answers from Erica's Expert" section of this chapter.) Instead, sprinkle baking soda on the floor and vacuum. Just don't do this around children with upper respiratory issues.

STORE PRODUCTS SAFELY

I also stopped storing cleaning products under the kitchen sink. Their bright candy colors can be too appealing to curious kids. (Always make sure the tops are tightly closed when using them around the house.) If you have to keep cleaning products in this area, use a baby-proof lock to keep the cabinet inaccessible to children or keep them in a container they can't open. I believe in storing these items away from food and high on a shelf or in a closet where they are difficult for kids to reach.

Think About Your Baby's Body Products

Before Arianna's chin started itching, I was using the products made for babies that are said to be gentle. But when I looked at their ingredients I saw chemicals and fragrances. (I thought it was interesting that someone actually thought these products were gentle for our babies!) So I sought out more gentle perfume- and chemical-free products. No scents. Nothing that could be an irritant when you inhaled it. Instead of lotions, I used coconut and olive oil for Arianna's body and hair, something my mother occasionally applied to mine and my sisters' hair when we were growing up. And I never used bubble bath, because of the ingredients (and the risk of possible urinary tract infections and irritation to the vagina). Plus, I was concerned about the long-term impact of bubble bath soap's chemicals.

From the day Arianna was born, I used a brand of chemical-free natural diapers. They're not as thick or as absorbent as popular brands of traditional diapers, so you have to change them more often, but they also don't have that smell that, although it's "baby fresh," is actually a chemical.

When Arianna was born, I didn't use baby wipes at home either. Instead, I'd use moistened cotton washcloths when I had to change her diaper. Then I'd take a tissue and pat her skin dry. To me, this was easier, because I didn't have to go to the store to buy more wipes. Also, using a washcloth was more cost-effective. With a newborn, I was doing lots of laundry anyway; what were a few small washcloths more?

Be Prepared!

Another way I've made our home healthy is to always be prepared for an emergency. Here are a few of the things I do.

FIRST AID

I keep a stocked first-aid kit in our home and take one with us when we travel. (If you have a car, I suggest you leave one in there, too. You never know when you're going to need one.) But I've added to it homeopathic items of my own. These include arnica gel, which is great for bumps and bruises; calendula ointment, for burns; and tea tree cream antiseptic, which you can use to clean out a cut. Also in there are Benadryl for allergic reactions, an EpiPen for serious allergic reactions, and our doctors' phone numbers.

EMERGENCY PHONE NUMBERS

Speaking of phone numbers, I keep a list of emergency phone numbers in a few places in my home, such as the bathroom medicine chests and in the kitchen. This is important in case I'm not home and a babysitter or relative is watching my kids. The list includes phone numbers for our doctors, the nearest hospital to our home, the hospital where the kids were born, the nearest relatives, and a close family friend. It's also important to have the local poison control number.

EPIPEN AWARENESS

I also have a poster that shows how to use an EpiPen, in case there's someone in our home who needs to use one on one of my children or on a guest but doesn't know how.

KID-PROOFING THE BATHROOM

I remember, as a kid, sneaking cough drops out of the bathroom and eating them like candy. There was medicine in them, but I didn't know that. All I knew was that they tasted good. That's why I make sure that anything in my kids' bathroom is absolutely safe. Why? The bathroom is often a place kids want to explore. There's something about the confined space and the different options where water is available—the toilet, sink, and bathtub—that's appealing to them. It's just too exciting and enticing. When my son was around four years old, he used to go in the bathroom, fill the sink with water, and make a pool for his superheroes. He'd pour in anything he could find. Luckily, all he was able to reach was liquid soap, toothpaste, and lotion, but with kids, anything can become a science experiment—and dangerous, because who knows what they're going to do with it?

IN CASE OF FIRE

I keep fire extinguishers in my home. I have one under the kitchen sink and one by the back door, where the washer and dryer are. Thankfully, we've never had to use ours, but you never know. I urge everyone to invest in fire extinguishers, whether you have children or not. Think about giving them away to a loved one as a gift. And regularly check their expiration dates.

ANSWERS FROM ERICA'S EXPERT

Jeffrey C. May is a certified indoor air quality professional (CIAQP) who got his MA in organic chemistry at Harvard University. He is the founder and principal scientist of May Indoor Air Investigations, a Massachusetts-based indoor air quality testing company that investigates mold and odor problems throughout the East Coast. He is also the author of *My House Is Killing Me!: The Home Guide for Families with Allergies and Asthma* and *My Office Is Killing Me!: The Sick Building Survival Guide*, and coauthor of *The Mold Survival Guide: For Your Home and for Your Health* and *Jeff May's Healthy Home Tips*. I wish I had known Jeff way back when Arianna had her chin irritation. But I met him much later on during this journey, when a doctor referred me to him. At the time, Addison's nose was really irritated because of particles in the air left over from a renovation at his school. Jeff's experience and insight are truly amazing.

A Healthier Home

What's the number one hidden threat to our health in our homes?

I would say concealed mold that's growing on dust in cooling systems or growing on dust in carpets placed on concrete. Even dead spores from mold on antique furniture that has been stored in a damp basement or garage can be a problem if disturbed. Few people suspect that mold growth can occur on dust captured in exposed fiberglass insulation in damp crawl spaces and basements, and this growth can also be a source of significant exposure to spores. Visible mold can be identified and eradicated, but invisible mold is difficult to identify, so you may continue to be exposed and suffer symptoms.

What type of health risk does mold pose? How do you know if you've got mold?

Some of the symptoms that my clients report to me include exacerbated asthma and allergy symptoms, chronic cough, headaches (often associated with sinus congestion), and fatigue. When mold is eliminated from their indoor environments, these clients usually report that their health has improved. A musty smell indicates that mold growth is present, but not all molds produce noticeable odors. This is why dust and possibly air testing, as part of a thorough professional walk-through, can be helpful.

What are the most toxic things we have in our homes?

Toxic chemicals can affect most cells and organs of anyone's body, whereas allergens affect only those people who have had previous exposure and become sensitized. And in any discussion of toxicity, we have to consider the exposure route: inhaling versus eating. Substances in our homes that are toxic if eaten include most cleaning products, pesticides, and paints. Some molds actually make mycotoxins (which are highly toxic chemicals), and there is no question that serious illness can result from eating certain moldy foods. Substances that are toxic if inhaled include carbon monoxide from a faulty heating system, strong solvent fumes, and smoke from a fire or even cigarettes. We all have different levels of sensitivity, however, so some of us react more strongly to environmental toxins. For example, people who have multiple chemical sensitivity (MCS) can experience brain fog and headaches from exposure to seemingly harmless concentrations of fragrances, fuel odors, combustion products, and pesticides.

Are there things many people think are healthy or not dangerous that are in fact dangerous?

Yes.

- Even "organic" food can have bacterial, fungal, or insect contaminants, especially if not stored properly.
- Aromatherapy introduces chemicals into the air that, even if from "natural" sources, still consist of potentially irritating and/or toxic substances. This includes essential oils, which are just organic chemicals not unlike, and in many cases identical to, those derived from petrochemicals.
- Jar candles create a cozy ambiance but produce soot particles that are unhealthy to breathe and that stain ceilings and walls.
- Ionizing air purifiers produce ozone, an irritating gas and one of the chief components of smog.
- Cool mist humidifiers can be contaminated with bacteria, yeast, or mold.
- Window and wall air conditioners and central air-conditioning systems can emit microbial allergens if not properly maintained.
- Sometimes the parents of a child with pet allergies will put a fish tank in the child's bedroom, as a substitute for a dog or cat. Air bubbling through the tank water can be a source of microbial and other allergens. In addition, highly allergenic dust mites can thrive occasionally on the tank cover, where they have abundant moisture and food if the fish flakes aren't carefully cleaned up.

What's the health risk of carpeting in children's bedrooms?

I've taken dust samples from hundreds of carpets, many of which were new, and have been amazed at the algae, mold, pet dander, yeast, and bacteria I've found in the dust. New carpets can be contaminated with microbial growth as a result of manufacturing techniques or storage practices. Some new carpets also "off-gas" toxic chemicals. (Off-gassing is the slow evaporation of chemicals or odors from a surface.) Even wool carpets can be hazardous if the fibers are deteriorating and producing high concentrations of microscopic wool fiber fragments that can cause coughing and eye irritation. A "used" carpet can contain pet allergens, mold, or bacteria due to prior spills, leaks, or nonprofessional cleaning. I prefer to see hard flooring in a child's bedroom, particularly if the child has allergies or asthma. You can always put a cotton area rug on the floor, and remove the rug for cleaning as needed.

What's the health risk of using carpet cleaner in a home where children live?

Children spend a lot of time on the floor, so their exposure to whatever is in the carpet is greater than an adult's exposure. Carpet cleaners are chemicals, which can leave residues. Carpets and pads can also become contaminated with microbial growth if they remain damp too long after being cleaned. Many parents try to save money by washing their own carpets. Rental equipment is never as efficient in removing moisture as professional carpet-cleaning equipment. Any carpet that stays damp for more than about a day and smells funky should be eliminated. You don't have to use chemicals to clean a carpet. You can treat carpeting with steam vapor, which can kill mites and fleas and destroy some allergens. The treatment, which is very different from "steam cleaning," doesn't leave behind a lot of moisture so the carpet dries quickly.

Is vacuuming a good or a bad idea when you have children with allergies/ asthma?

Dust is the devil for allergy and asthma sufferers, so it is extremely important to minimize dust levels in the entire house, particularly in a child's bedroom. It's essential, however, to use a HEPA (high-efficiency particulate arrestance) vacuum, preferably with a bag. If your vacuum is bag-less, be sure to empty the dust container outdoors. Don't forget to vacuum under and behind furniture. Energetic vacuuming stirs up dust, so move the floor nozzle slowly across a carpet's surface. Studies have shown that repeated passes are more effective in dust removal, so vacuum thoroughly for several minutes, going back and forth repeatedly over an area. Keep in mind that you can never remove all the dust from a carpet. If your child is particularly sensitive to dust, he or she should not be present in the room you are vacuuming. If weather permits, you can open a window in the room or put a fan in the window on "Exhaust," so disturbed dust will be carried on airflows to the exterior.

What about paint and wallpaper—do they pose any health risk? What are the best paints to use in your home?

The best paints are those that are water-based and that have low emission rates of volatile organic compounds (VOCs). If you want to be sure about the emissions from a particular paint, get a sample and paint it on a piece of scrap wood. Let the paint dry and see if it smells after a day or two. It's probably not a good idea to use wallpaper in bathrooms, because high humidity can lead to mold growth on the paper or paste. Vinyl wallpaper can also be a concern in air-conditioned buildings that are located in hot and humid climates. Moisture can be trapped behind the wallpaper, which can lead to hidden mold growth and musty odors.

What's the best idea for cleaning surfaces that babies and toddlers touch and eat off, such as their toys, high chair tray, and crib railing?

Any detergent intended for surface cleaning, and water, is fine. Lots of people like to clean with vinegar, but I don't like the odor. After washing a surface, be sure to rinse it off and then dry it. Avoid fragranced wipes that can leave a residue. It's better to use paper towels or rags you can wash frequently rather than a sponge, which can become infested with bacteria. If a sponge smells "sour" due to bacterial growth, it will leave a sour smell on the surface. Last, don't forget to clean one of the surfaces that toddlers frequently touch and eat food from: your own hands.

Why is it a good idea to take our shoes off at the door?

Foot traffic can bring pollen, mold, lawn pesticides, and even lead dust into a home. The soil immediately around older homes can contain high levels of lead from old exterior paint and from trucks and cars that ran on lead-containing gasoline. Removing shoes at the door not only helps keep your house cleaner, but also reduces your exposure to exterior allergens and toxins.

Is there a health risk to having too many electric things plugged into our rooms?

The biggest risks from the use of electricity are fire and shocks. Power cords should never run under rugs or be in contact with electric baseboard heaters. Floor outlets can be dangerous, because if a paper clip or something else that's metal falls into the outlet, it can cause a short and start a fire. Young children who crawl or play on a floor will have ready access to a floor outlet. That's why all outlets within a child's reach should have child-safe covers on them. Some studies claim that exposure to low levels of electromagnetic fields (EMF) cause health symptoms, but in the scientific community, this assertion is very controversial.

Are there typical, store-bought, traditional cleaning products in our homes that pose a danger to us?

If you or anyone in your household has asthma or any other respiratory condition, it's best to avoid using solvent-based cleaners or cleaners with strong odors, including fragrances. Any time products such as these are used, keep windows open for ventilation. Anyone sensitive to the products should not be present when they are being used. It's best not to use aerosol cans, which spread chemicals into the air. Be careful about mixing certain cleaning products. Anything that contains bleach should not be mixed with a product that contains ammonia. If these chemicals are mixed, a toxic gas is produced.

What are the healthiest ways to clean your house and clothes?

- Clean often, at least once a week, and avoid fragranced cleaning products.
- Use a HEPA vacuum for all household cleaning, because conventional vacuums emit allergens and irritants in their exhaust.
- If you hire cleaners to clean your home, never allow them to use their own vacuum in your house; otherwise, your house could become contaminated with pet dander and mold spores from someone else's home.
- Dust surfaces carefully and keep a window open for ventilation.
- If you have allergies or asthma, wear a disposable, two-strap NIOSH-approved N95 mask when cleaning. (NIOSH is the National Institute for Occupational Safety and Health.) Single-strap and hospital masks that loop around the ears are not adequate.
- Families with allergies and asthma should not wash clothing with laundry detergents that contain enzymes, which can exacerbate asthma symptoms. Always check the label for ingredients, even if the product is labeled "natural" or "organic."
- Don't use fabric softener sheets in the dryer because the sheets leave chemical residues on clothing that can be irritating to people who are sensitized.
- Clean upholstered furniture with a HEPA vacuum; then treat with steam vapor; that is, do not steam clean. For folks with allergies, leather is best.

What's the number one store-bought chemical that we ought not to bring into our homes?

In a word, pesticides. This includes mothballs, bee and wasp sprays, and even some potting soil. Don't keep soil that contains pesticides or herbicides in your basement or attached garage, because air flows from these spaces into your habitable rooms.

Is a wood floor that has a polyurethane finish dangerous or toxic?

The off-gassing from polyurethane finish depends on the solvent. Water-based finishes tend to be less of a problem. The emissions from a solvent-based coating (which is harder than the water based) can take a few days to off-gas, but usually are not a problem. I did have a big problem with a rapid-dry urethane finish in my kitchen that took a month to off-gas. I could not go into the kitchen and had to have two box fans running 24-7, one on "Supply" and the other on "Exhaust," with the kitchen sealed off from the rest of the house.

What's the most priceless piece of information that parents need to know about keeping their homes healthy?

Control the relative humidity (RH) in your home. In most climates, if the RH gets above 50 percent in a crawl space or unfinished basement, above 60 percent in a finished basement, or above 80 percent in rooms above ground level, you might be heading for mold-growth problems. And where there is mold growth, there are usually mold-eating mites and other insects that flourish in high humidity. These creatures produce allergenic fecal material. House dust mites also need moisture to survive, so controlling the RH helps to control dust mite populations. When we sleep, we introduce moisture into our mattresses, pillows, and bedding with our bodies and our breath. Another way to avoid dust mite exposure is to put dust mite encasings on all mattresses, box springs, and pillows. Use the encasings with polyurethane liners, which helps keep the moisture we produce out of the mattress and pillows.

Is it a problem to inhale these polyurethane liners?

In my experience these liners are not a problem with respect to off-gassing. On the other hand, I have seen cotton encasings that were not effective due to excessive pore size between the fibers (which allows mite allergens to escape a contaminated mattress). In addition, the porous liners, whether polyester or cotton, allow moisture to enter the mattress. Thus, if there is a mite colony, it lives on forever with the body moisture supplied. The polyurethane coating prevents most of the moisture from entering the mattress. Less expensive liners can be used on a box spring.

Is there a risk to sending your clothes to the dry cleaner because of the chemicals they use?

For most people there is little risk. For those who are chemically sensitized, the off-gassing can be problematic, so you should hang clothing that has been dry-cleaned in a room that is well ventilated to the exterior (for a few days). An alternative to standard dry cleaning with PERC (perchloroethylene) is liquid carbon dioxide. This is very "green" and there are a few shops around that use it.

If you suffer from seasonal allergies, should you keep your windows closed or open?

This is the conundrum if you have allergies. There are, however, some fans equipped with filters, and these can be used (so long as the filter is kept dry). It's best to know what allergens are in the air (grass or tree pollen, mold, etc.) and to keep the windows shut when the personal allergens are present outdoors.

Chapter 6

Thriving at School

If we moms and dads don't advocate for our children, no one else will. You have to raise a ruckus and never stop. When the school sees me coming they roll their eyes and brace themselves, because here comes "Hurricane Holly"! I love that because they know they can't roll over me. I am doing my job! Push fear out of the way and focus on the fact that if you don't speak up, your child will suffer. Time is not on our side, so sitting on the sidelines is not an option. If you keep that in your mind, your inner momma bear will come out of hibernation and awaken and then watch out. Martin Luther King said, "Our lives begin to end the day we become silent about things that matter."

—Holly Robinson Peete, mother of four

My son was about to enter his first year of preschool when we found out that he had asthma and more than a dozen food allergies. Addison was diagnosed with cold-induced asthma, which meant that the cold weather triggered symptoms such as coughing spells. I thought this might be a potential problem during roof time, which was his preschool's equivalent of recess. (Because we live in New York City, the kids at his school went up on the roof to play, rather than to a playground, as they do at some schools.) But then I thought, *How much running could he do in such a confined space as a small roof?*

Addison was fine in the early fall, but once November rolled around he was coughing and sick every time he went outside. I started sending him to school with a scarf to wear during roof time, to cover up his mouth, but when that didn't help I didn't know what to do. This was a new situation for me. (Though Arianna had gone to the same preschool, this had not been an issue for her.) *I guess he needs to stay inside during roof time,* I thought. When I told his teachers this, they looked at me as if I were speaking a foreign language. So I went to speak to the director of the school.

"My son has cold-induced asthma," I explained. "He's got to stay inside during roof time."

The director shook her head no. "All children this age need to get physical and play outdoors for a certain amount of time each day," she said. "It's a New York State law."

"That may apply to those kids over there," I said, pointing to a group of children gathered on the rug. "But my child has a health condition. He can't go out when it's twenty degrees." While I was talking, the school director continued to shake her head no. She acted as if I were one of those overbearing parents who just didn't want her child to go outside because it was cold. And I could tell from her reaction that she had dealt with plenty of those parents; she was armed and ready. But I wasn't trying to be bossy or pick a fight; I was trying to protect my son's health.

Despite my protests, the school refused to comply with my request. I even offered to come to Addison's class during roof time each day and sit with him so it would not be an inconvenience to the teachers. No luck. I spent that whole winter upset and complaining about this, but nothing changed. By the time warm weather rolled around I was relieved, because the cold-induced asthma was not much of a concern during this time, but I was also very disappointed with the school because of their lack of awareness and action.

At the end of August during the summer before Addison's second year at that preschool, I received a call from his best friend's mother. School was starting in September, the day after Labor Day, and this mom was concerned. Her son had recently been diagnosed with asthma and he wasn't supposed to go out in the cold either. Knowing all that I'd gone through the previous year on this issue, she nervously asked me, "What are we going to do with our boys at school?" My first thought was, *What is the school going to do? Isn't it their responsibility?* That year, I waited to see if the cold was still a problem for Addison, hoping that he'd outgrown it. But when brisk temperatures arrived in New York City, so did Addison's coughing fits. Obviously his lungs weren't able to endure the cold at that particular point in his life. I'd had enough. I went to the director once again.

"This is my son's health we're talking about," I said. "He needs to stay inside during roof time. Tell me what I *need* to do to make this happen."

"We need to know there's a medical reason why he can't go outside," the director said. "You need a doctor's note."

Say no more, I thought. It had never dawned on me to get a doctor's note.

I called the pediatrician that day. She actually had to write a prescription saying that my son was not supposed to be exposed to cold air or to play outside in any temperature below sixty degrees. However, this wasn't the end of the issue.

"What are we going to do with him?" one teacher asked.

"This is for you to work out," I said. "He's in your care." After all, my son may have been the first kid in their school who was unable to go out in the cold weather, but he certainly wasn't going to be the last. I was just opening up the door for the others. *They'd better come up with a plan*, I thought. And eventually they did. Some days, Addison sat in the director's office reading books or drawing; other times, a teacher stayed with him in the classroom. The teachers weren't happy about it. It was an inconvenience during a time when they wanted to take a break or get the room ready for the next activity. I understood that. But this was a health issue we were dealing with, and without his health, all that other stuff was irrelevant. (A side note: by Addison's second year, that other boy was inside with him during roof time, for the same reason; by his third year, there were four other kids who needed to stay inside.)

Unfortunately, that wasn't the only time I struggled to get my point across at my kids' schools. One day, the nurse at my daughter's former elementary school told me that she wasn't able to give Arianna the homeopathic brand of cough medicine I had sent to school. *Why?* I thought. *Is it because it's from a health food store and not a drugstore?* The nurse went on to say that she didn't recognize the brand and wasn't trained to give it. She said, "I'll do it this one time, but cannot do it again." This didn't make sense, because I had a prescription from our pediatrician telling her exactly how much of the medicine to give my daughter. Despite this, the nurse was saying no to something my child needed. All I kept thinking was how behind the times this nurse appeared to be, especially in the twenty-first century, when more and more people were turning to homeopathic and alternative remedies. It was her resistance to this, and lack of awareness as a school nurse, that bothered me.

I also had to fight for my daughter to bring her own lunch to school, because as I've mentioned, at this particular school the children were required to eat the cafeteria food. At the time, the majority of this food was highly processed, and many items were made with sugar (one being jelly sandwiches on white bread!). There were two reasons I wanted Arianna to bring her own lunch, besides the fact that she had a nut allergy. In kindergarten, she came home almost daily complaining of stomachaches. At first I thought it was nerves; after all, she was at a new school, and kindergarten was very different from preschool. But the stomachaches continued for weeks, well past the point where I knew she was acclimated, comfortable, and happy at school. I asked her what she was eating for lunch and she told me about the bagels she ate *every day*. I didn't think much of it at first. After all, bagels are dry and seemingly harmless—or so I thought until I took her to see Dr. Pescatore because of her stomach. He asked her about the foods she ate often, and she told him about the bagels.

"She's getting too much wheat, gluten, and yeast," he said. "Of course her stomach hurts."

At this point we were just coming off the summer when Addison was in the hospital. So, to me, a plain, dry bagel seemed like a better option than the meat served at school, something I had told Arianna not to eat. But once Dr. Pescatore made me aware of the issue with all those bagels, I went to Arianna's kindergarten teacher and asked if my daughter could bring her own lunch to school.

"She's only eating bagels because there's nothing else she likes to eat," I explained. I even went on to tell her about our summer and the horrible bacteria that had landed Addison on an operating table for emergency surgery.

But the teacher shook her head no. "The school's policy is that no outside food is brought in," she said. This made no sense to me, especially since food is brought in frequently for birthdays, class celebrations, and special days such as Multicultural Day. After this, I went to talk to the school nurse. I was just trying to gather information and get some answers. But she told me the same thing the teacher had. "Take it up with the head of the lower school if you want," she suggested. So I did.

I sat in that woman's office crying as I shared my story about the devastating experience Addison had had with the nasty, life-threatening bacteria. The head of the lower school was kind and sympathetic, but she still didn't care that I wanted Arianna to bring her own lunch to school. The excuse she gave me was that the school was concerned that kids would leave food in their lockers and this would cause a rodent problem. *Really? Is this the best you can tell me?* I thought. Other schools weren't afraid, and this school *did* have food in the building. What they didn't have in place was a system to allow kids to bring their food in and teach them how to throw it out properly, as they were doing with the current cafeteria food. Also, many children had after-school snacks in their lockers anyway. (I know mine did.)

The problem was not rodents; it was red tape. And that's what I said. I wasn't putting the school down, but I was frustrated with the lack of awareness in the nutritional area—especially in these modern times, and at a progressive school. To me, the issue didn't seem to be rodents, but the bottom line: the decision was being made by someone looking at a spreadsheet rather than thinking about our children.

I must have gotten on the kindergarten teacher's nerves with all my talk about the school food, because when I spoke to her next, she said, "Why don't you just join the food committee?"

There's a food committee? I thought. *Now I'm getting somewhere.*

I was excited. If the kids couldn't bring their own lunches to school maybe we could at least improve what they were being served. Unfortunately, my excitement was short-lived. When I joined the food committee, their big goal was getting bagels off the menu. This was not because they were unhealthy, but because the other moms were worried about their kids gaining weight from eating only bagels for lunch and having more than one bagel at a time. Once I found out about the committee, I attended the only two meetings they had. Why only two? Because once they'd successfully gotten rid of the bagels, they also got rid of the food committee. After that no one really cared about the food that was being served.

Despite my efforts, there has not been a food committee since. When I asked the school about creating one and someone guided me to the parent association, their response to me was "We have no plans at this time to have a food committee." Yes, I thought about forming a group of my own and having like-minded moms come to my home or meet to discuss food issues at school. But we had no one to take our issues to. Who was available to listen when it was not a priority at the school? What was more of a concern was bettering the math and science program, for example; health was not on their radar. We'd have had no support.

One day shortly after this, Arianna came home asking me if she could try the school's chicken nuggets. "Please, Mom," she begged. "Everyone eats them, and they look so good!" Obviously after my summer with Addison I was wary of a lot of foods, especially when I had no idea where the school's meat came from. But after enough begging, I finally said yes.

Well, we both learned a lesson when she came down with five days of diarrhea right after eating them. I told the school nurse about this, and asked if there were any other kids out of school for the same reason. Her response? "A stomach bug is going around." But Arianna hadn't had a fever or any other symptoms of a stomach bug. This wasn't a stomach bug; it was a food bug.

That was it for me. Once again I thought, *Enough is enough. I have to listen to that little voice inside of me.* I had control over my child's food at home and I wanted control when she was at school. Again I went to talk to the school nurse and the head of school to discuss Arianna bringing her own lunch. But this time, I didn't ask for their permission. Instead I said, "What do I *need* to do for Arianna to bring her own lunch to school?"

"There needs to be a medical reason why she can't eat the school lunch," the head of the lower school told me.

The doctor's note again! I called Dr. Pescatore, who had diagnosed the reason for Arianna's stomachaches (which, by the way, ceased when the bagels were off the school menu). He wrote a note, but it took a few rewrites until the school accepted it, because the note needed to detail what might happen if Arianna ate their food, the potential side effects, the medical reason, and so on. (This seemed to have become a game, with me pitted against the entire school administration.) Finally, the note worked for them, and after a lot of tears, frustration, and red tape, my daughter had the school's permission to bring her lunch from home.

Once they got the note, the school told me that if Arianna was not allowed to eat the school's lunch, she was also not allowed to take part in any communal celebration or eat anything else at school. She wasn't able to have candy if the science teacher passed it out as a surprise, or cupcakes if another child brought them in for a birthday celebration. I was really disappointed by this—not the fact that she was not able to eat these foods, but at the school's actually thinking it was okay to ostracize a child due to health issues. The doctor's note had explained specifically what Arianna was able to eat. Still, the school was banning her from everything and making no helpful suggestions for how to include her.

After that, I had to bring Arianna's own stash of treats and ask the teacher to give them to her when another child came in with a treat for the class. I also asked the teacher to let me know in advance when the class was going to celebrate a child's birthday with treats brought in by parents. This way I could send an appropriate treat in with Arianna. I didn't ask the school to make the treat for her, to supply her with the treat, to use their kitchen to bake it, or even to warm it up; all I asked for was a date. This seemed like an easy request, since these events were scheduled well in advance.

At first the teacher said yes, but once she'd discussed it with the school administration, they said it was too much work and that she was unable to notify me. I was speechless and in shock.

I had no problem with the fact that I needed proper and official backing to allow Addison to stay inside during roof time or to allow Arianna to bring her own lunch. But once I got this backing, I handled it carefully. I made sure to photocopy those notes and had them put in my children's files at the doctor's office in case we needed a new note the following year or for any other reason. I also photocopied one for myself and kept it in a special school file in my home. My advice is to save these kinds of documents and never throw them out, in case the school loses them or a similar issue arises. (This was several years ago, and I still have all my notes and documentation even though we have since switched schools.) Have the school and your doctor sign your copy and date it. If it's an e-mail, print it out, because computers can crash. You have to have that hard copy to back yourself up.

I didn't do all this because I'm some wacky mom who obsesses over her kids (though I am sure it looked that way to some people who didn't know the details of our situation). I didn't do it because my children asked me to. I didn't do it to try to give the school a hard time. (After all, having Arianna bring her lunch from home was only more work for me, because I had to prepare it each morning.) I did it because my children's health is important to me. It comes first. We are our children's voices when they're young and can't speak up for themselves. And in certain situations, we are all they have. If we're not standing up for our own kids, then who is? No one. We can't be afraid to be vocal. It's like being a customer in a restaurant. If you're not satisfied with the service or the meal, you're going to say something. When it comes to your kids' schools, it should be no different. This is where your child spends most of her day. This is where she's learning. Schools wouldn't be schools without the kids and the parents. We make the difference. So you can sit back and watch, or you can help make your child's school better, more aware, and evolved.

To be clear, I don't mean that we need to go in and handicap our children by handling every school issue for them. For example, one day Arianna was late to school because she had had an early morning doctor's appointment. She was upset about missing school because she had homework to hand in for one of the classes. When we got upstairs, we saw that her teacher was conducting another class.

"Mom, will you go in there and give her my homework?" Arianna asked nervously.

"I don't go to this school," I said. "It's not my homework. I already finished fourth grade."

I understood that Arianna didn't want to interrupt the teacher, and do so in front of a full class, but this was her issue. I encouraged her to go in there and turn it in.

"Just go into that classroom and tell her you're sorry for interrupting, but that you were at an appointment," I told her. After all, she needs to know how to communicate in that situation. "You can do it. If you can make a horse jump you can go in there and do this!" I said, referring to her competitive horseback riding skills.

Soon enough, Arianna had worked up the nerve and gone into that classroom. She survived the nervousness, and I think it gave her a little boost of self-confidence to tackle something she was afraid of, to see that everything had worked out okay, and that it was better than she imagined.

But when it comes to other things—big issues such as our children's health—then your voice matters. It matters whether you're at a private school or a public school. It matters whether you're paying full tuition or are on financial aid. There was a point at both of the schools I talk about here where I was pretty sure I was the mom who was the headache. But I didn't care. I was the one taking my kids to the doctors' offices. I was the one who had to care for them when they were sick. I was the one who was drained, exhausted. I was the one thinking outside the box. I was the one who knew I was not too old or too good to learn and become more aware. I was the one learning something from each doctor's appointment we went to.

A lot of times we as moms and dads don't feel we have a choice. But we *do*. We have a choice in everything. We just have to be proactive. I'm certainly not saying do everything for your kids. Or make a big deal of things that don't need to be a big deal. I'm saying help them—especially when it's health related.

I once heard about a kindergartener at my son's former school who came down with the chicken pox. Another child in the class hadn't been vaccinated so the school called the parents of the child who had not been vaccinated and told them she had to stay home from school for three weeks to make sure she didn't get this disease. That really got me thinking. *Did they also close the entire school and fumigate it for the chicken pox virus?* No. The child who had chicken pox had already been all over the school. She had touched the library books, the railing on the stairs, items in the gym, and many other things throughout the school. Her germs were there. The school had already been exposed. If the unvaccinated child's parents didn't mind their child attending the school, then why did the school mind?

We do not tell the healthy kids to stay home from school when strep throat goes around. Rather than reacting when kids get sick, schools ought to be protecting our kids' health. Schools need to know that our children's health is a priority. I want to start a movement. I want these schools to hear the parents. Because this goes beyond health. It affects our kids and their self-esteem. For example, if a school is not nut-free, children with nut allergies may have to sit at a separate table, and risk being ostracized by their peers. Maybe some kids do not mind this, but others will, and it sets these kids up for bullying. Worse yet, they may feel the school is on the side of the bullies. I'm not saying that every school has to be peanut-free, but parents should be aware of what they can do to protect their kids emotionally, too. Use common sense and don't wait for the worst to happen before making changes. Learn to become more aware. It's easy, and it's free.

ANSWERS FROM ERICA'S EXPERT

If you're lucky, you go through school and find that one teacher—the teacher who believes in you, encourages you, and inspires you. She becomes that teacher you simply can't forget, the one whose lessons go beyond the classroom and live on well past your school years. For me that was my fifth-grade teacher, Jan Schlossberg. My sister, who is just twelve months younger than I, was in Mrs. Schlossberg's fifth grade the following year and felt the same way. This woman was magical to us. She didn't do anything extra for me, and I wasn't the teacher's pet. (Although I so wanted to be.) But she made me feel safe, secure, comfortable, nurtured, and confident. I knew she cared for me and wanted the best for me. She was rooting for me without rooting for me. (All that and beautiful, too, as glamorous as Susan Lucci—the epitome of glamour to us kids at the time—with her hair, makeup, and nails always done.) Neither my sister nor I ever forgot Mrs. Schlossberg. Even as adults, on April 30 each year, we'll call each other and one of us will say, "Happy birthday, Mrs. Schlossberg." (The only other person's birthday we used to call each other on was Michael Jackson's, on August 29, so that gives you a sense of the high regard in which we hold Mrs. Schlossberg.) It became a game to see who would call the other first. Even better, though, is that we now get to call, e-mail, or send flowers directly to Mrs. Schlossberg since she is in our lives today as a friend and still as a teacher.

As adults, my sister and I tried to track her down for years, with no luck. Then one day, my sister was home from work with the flu and decided to try again. This time she succeeded, and we were finally connected, via telephone—twenty-eight years after we were in her class! When my sister and I shared with her what she had meant to us, she said she had no idea that she had had this impact on us. Today, Mrs. Schlossberg is still a teacher, and I know she has a lot of wisdom to impart after three decades of teaching. I heard that a parent referred to her as the "child whisperer." She knows not only how to teach and be what a child needs and deserves, but she knows how to keep effective parent-teacher dialogue open. She is just an amazing teacher and when I refer to her I can honestly say, I had the BEST teacher EVER! Here Jan Schlossberg, mother of two sons, shares some of that expertise.

Dealing with Schools

What's an effective way for parents to communicate with teachers and school administration in an open dialogue?

Communication should be the hallmark of any school. Back-to-school night and parent-teacher conferences are the official means of communication. However, if there are parental or teacher concerns, an additional conference should be scheduled. Parents always have the right to meet and confer with the teachers and administrative staff. Since the teacher has firsthand knowledge of the child, it is always preferable that parents express their concerns with the teacher first. If the problem continues, then it is proper protocol to bring in an administrator for continued dialogue.

Why is it so important for parents to be involved with their kids' school and their education?

It has been said that it "takes a village to raise a child." Parental involvement is essential for the child's growth. Each school will have its own policy about parental involvement. It is my opinion, however, that schools that encourage parent involvement help create a vested interest in the school. When I was in graduate school, one of my professors said, "Schools will always rise to the level of the parent's expectations." Good schools already do this, but schools should always be open to parental input.

What are the best ways for parents to get involved with their kids' school and their education?

Board of Education monthly meetings, parent association meetings, and volunteering in the classroom are excellent ways to get involved. I feel that parent meetings and involvement in the classroom are equally important. The parent meetings help you understand the global picture for the month. Working in the classroom helps you observe both the teacher and your child. Elementary teachers always have tremendous amounts of cutting, drawing, sorting, and coloring to do. Every teacher will always be grateful for help with these tasks. Working parents may not have the flexibility to participate during the day, but they can take material home to help prepare for an activity. The child sees this involvement, and it makes her feel important.

What is the first step to take if your child is having a problem with a teacher at school?

I cannot emphasize this enough. Begin with the teacher. If this problem involves a particular teacher, he/she should be given the opportunity to address the problem first. If the problem continues, then it is important to bring an administrator into the mix.

What are some of the biggest mistakes parents make in dealing with their child's teacher/school?

When a parent makes the teacher an adversary rather than an advocate, teachers can become defensive. Most teachers love children and are passionate about creating a good learning environment. They want the child to be successful under their watch. If the parent goes into "attack mode," then dialogue becomes slanted and difficult. If the parent or teacher expresses a concern, and the issue is dealt with directly, without accusations or anger, then resolution can be achieved. Teachers have the same need to please as any other professional. They want their students to succeed.

What can a parent do if a child cries every day before going to school and says he or she does not want to go? How can you deal with your child in that case?

It is so important to bring the teacher into the loop. Communicate with the teacher immediately. Often he or she can solve the problem easily and quickly. If the problem persists, do not give up. Let the teacher know. It may also be advisable to bring the child into this conversation. Persistence and diligence are noble qualities. Parents will always be their child's best advocate. I advocated for my sons until they were able to speak for themselves. Teachers also want the best for the child. Letting the child know that you are there to support him is crucial. Your child needs to know that he is not alone with this problem. Be honest. Tell your child that you are there to support and help him. If a young child is not able to articulate the problem, then you still need to communicate with the teacher. Teachers are trained to understand young children, and should be able to identify the problem.

How can you deal with the school if your child has a food allergy or other health issue?

Before school begins, parents are asked to complete a health form. Complete this form carefully. Then, prior to school beginning, ask for a conference with the teacher and the school nurse specifically to address the issue. It is important for a teacher to know about food allergies. If the child is allergic to grass, flowers, and plants, the teacher and health office need to know. They also need to know what medications or treatments should be used in case the child has a reaction. Being proactive is crucial.

If the child is a vegan, it is important to inform the school. Before the winter holiday and Valentine's Day parties, I always informed my students' parents and let them bring in a vegan alternative to the cupcake.

If there is a problem related to how someone's child is doing in class and they do not want to wait until conference time to address it, what are your suggestions for rectifying the issue?

Communication is the key. If a problem develops before the scheduled conference period, it is imperative to let the teacher know. You can do this with a simple call or e-mail. If you feel like you need a face-to-face conference, then it is your right to schedule one. Never be afraid to question a teacher about an issue. Part of her job is to communicate with you. Teachers want parents to be happy with their child's development.

Kids sometimes are seen as not telling the truth or including all the important facts related to things that happen at school with a teacher. What advice do you have with this situation?

This is a slippery slope problem. Imagine the adult teacher's credibility being pitted against that of a five-year-old. With that said, I have always told parents that if they believe part of what their child says about the teacher, I will believe a part of what is said about that teacher. Before a parent overreacts to what a child has told them about a specific situation, it is imperative to talk with the teacher. I am not suggesting that the child's credibility be questioned, but a child's imagination can often change the details and facts of a situation. So before you go down that road, it is important to bring the facts of the problem to the teacher.

What is your feeling about children being rewarded with candy or other treats from their teachers?

As part of the daily routine, I am hesitant to reward my students with a candy treat. First of all, I don't like to reward good learning with sugar. Stickers, awards, and peer recognition are good alternatives to sugar rewards. However, once in a great while, I will reward the children with a small sugar treat. For example, during Halloween, I might give a child one candy corn. During Valentine's Day, I could give my students one small candy heart. This will typically take place prior to our holiday party. Mostly, though, I prefer to keep food separate from learning as a reward.

Is there anything you have noticed that helps a child who does not sit still or can't focus while at school?

A child who may be developmentally immature may need some extra attention. Often a sticker program solves this problem. This technique is called behavior modification. Always involve the parents with this approach. For example, if the child had a difficult day listening and working cooperatively, then the parent will become aware of this. A chart plus a small note goes home with the child at the close of the day. Often I will either call or e-mail the parent about what transpired during the day. My belief is that if the parents are on board, then you are working as a team. I ask my parents to have a "conversation" with their child about the day, to define what happened and suggest what alternative behavioral choices could have been made. When the child receives an agreed-upon number of happy face days, he can be rewarded with an inexpensive toy or book. If the problem persists, a different approach may be needed. For example, if a child is being consistently impulsive, we can work with a behavior chart designed specifically for impulsivity. If the child did not have a successful day, then I might suggest that a "consequence" is appropriate. I like to use the word *consequence*. As humans we must always face consequences for a particular choice. I think that a child as young as five years old can learn what the word *consequence* means. It is holding the child accountable for his behavior. The behavior chart will be designed to deal specifically with the child's issues. More severe problems, such as ADHD (attention deficit hyperactivity disorder) may require the help of a pediatrician. Controlling the child's diet can often help with this particular issue.

Do you think a child's diet has anything to do with her ability to stay focused and remain calm while at school?

Absolutely. Each child needs a good breakfast of protein, carbohydrates, and some fruit. Their midmorning snack should include cheese, fruit, and a few crackers. Lunch should, once again, include protein, a carbohydrate, a vegetable, and fruit. Children work hard and play hard. The protein and carbohydrates give them the fuel they need to focus and learn.

Do you feel teachers can do more to help prevent bullying during school hours? If so, what can they do?

Bullying is a problem that plagues most American schools. I believe that most teachers have had many in-service workshops about this topic. Each school should have a no-bullying policy. There should be zero tolerance for this type of behavior. Teachers can begin this discussion with preschool children. After the discussion, the children can create posters about bullies, puppets for role-playing, and written stories in journals. These are just a few of the ideas used to support the notion that bullying in any form is hurtful, wrong, and simply unacceptable. Cyber bullying is another version of this behavior. There should also be zero tolerance for this hurtful behavior. Teachers need to give their students strategies for handling a bully. These strategies should include techniques for protecting yourself, peer help and support, and immediate teacher help.

Respect seems to be diminishing in so many schools today across the globe. Do you think it has anything to do with the fact that our children are addressing their teachers by their first names rather than more formally, as in Mrs. Schlossberg or Ms. Jan?

I cannot teach without respect. Before a teacher demands respect, however, she has to show her students what respect means. First of all, I am always respectful toward my students. I will always say "please" before I ask them to do something and "thank you" once they have responded. I celebrate each minute with them for being the remarkable little people they are in this world. In my room, we have the Magic X. This is simply colorful tape on our carpet in the form of an X. If a child has responded to a question, he will be asked to stand on the Magic X. We then blow kisses of appreciation toward that child. This idea comes from a wonderful educator, Michael Brandwein. He believes that you have to treat the child respectfully before you can ask to be treated respectfully yourself. I cannot ask for respect simply because I am a teacher. My job is to demonstrate respect over and over and over again until it becomes automatic to my young charges. The Magic X might not be appropriate for older students, but the concept can be used. I also speak in soft whispers to my students. I tell them repeatedly that "words are powerful." If I softly ask a child to stop doing a particular action, the words should be loud inside his brain. This is all part of teaching respect. Although I may be a bit old-fashioned about being addressed as Mrs. Schlossberg, I do not believe that calling me by my first name will take away from the respect I insist upon receiving. I share my humanity with my students. I let them know what feels good and what is hurtful. I try to role-play and model the type of behavior I want to encourage. When I want my students' attention, my presence alone should be enough for them to stop what they are doing. No words, no loud shouts—just me. That is respect at its best.

If you have a choice as to which school to send your child to, what should you look for when researching schools?

Every parent should ask lots of pertinent questions. The answers you receive should help guide you in your school decision. You should also ask for a school tour while school is in session. Look at the children there. Do they seem engaged? Do they appear happy? Is the room colorful? Does it look magical? Does it have the children's work displayed in a meaningful way? Would you be happy in this type of classroom? Does the room look inviting? Do the teachers appear happy and engaged? Most schools have a mission statement that explicitly states what the school is about. For example, a school that focuses more on the humanities—writing, literature, history, art, and music—will often state this in its mission statement. Traditional schools will approach learning in more traditional ways. This is more of a serious approach. It is very effective for a certain type of child. Religious schools will teach ethics and values based on specific doctrines. The job of parents is to think about what they value as a family. Does the school support your family and personal values? If it does, then it will be a good match.

How do you know if your child is having a problem at school? What are the signs to look for?

If your child is unable to articulate a problem, look for signs of stress. For example, a normally compliant child will suddenly become moody and oppositional. The child may exhibit difficulty sleeping or will wake up during the night. Not wanting to eat and loss of appetite are often signs of stress. Sometimes I will ask a young child to draw a picture of herself in her classroom. This can serve as a springboard for discussion. When you see signs of stress, communicate with your child's teacher immediately. Express your concerns and together work on figuring out how to solve the problem.

Chapter 7

Traveling with Children

When I travel with my kids, I give them as much info about what we're doing as possible. It gives them a sense of being in charge. To keep the kids entertained, I really like old-fashioned toys. Crayons, pencils, Etch A Sketch, and books on tape are a big winner for our family. Trips are a time to unplug and relax. It takes the kids a minute to adjust from the busy Internet world we live in, but once they do, it's wonderful to watch their imaginations unfold.

—Veronica Webb, mother of two

Once, when Arianna was six years old and Addison was four, the three of us and my mother went to Miami, Florida. When we got to the airport and off the plane, we headed to the bathroom. (That's one of my top travel rules: always have the kids use the bathroom when you see one.) As soon as we entered the bathroom, I noticed that an airport custodian was mopping the floor with a bright, bubble gum pink cleaning liquid that had a very strong chemical scent. Within seconds, Addison said, "It stinks in here." Then the coughing spell started. He was coughing like crazy. He'd obviously inhaled fumes from that pink cleaning stuff and they were interfering with his breathing. This went on for several minutes, even after we'd rushed out of the bathroom. I tried giving him water, but that didn't work.

Then we headed outside to get into the rental car. Once inside, I rolled down the window, thinking that fresh air was what Addison needed. It wasn't. The coughing continued and wasn't getting better. Finally, I gave him a puff of the asthma inhaler I carry with us for emergencies—especially when we travel. I've probably used it a handful of times in his life, and I don't like doing so, but in this particular situation I felt I had no choice. We were in a city that was not our own hometown, and Addison was having a coughing fit. I certainly wasn't going to risk my child's health when nothing else was working. After the puff of the inhaler, he was a little better, though still coughing.

At this point, I was a bit nervous. My heart was racing. I tried to think positively, but at the same time I was hoping and praying that this trip to Miami would not include a visit to the emergency room. We drove around looking for a health food store, and I was thrilled when I spotted a Whole Foods. Leaving the kids in the car with my mother, I ran inside and started looking for things I thought would help us, such as eucalyptus essential oil. (I say "us" because Addison was not alone. Though he was the one physically affected, the rest of us were affected emotionally. We were all in this together.)

After I'd grabbed the essential oil, we were blessed again when I spotted a big-box store in the same shopping plaza as the Whole Foods. In there I bought a vaporizer. Back in the car, I had Addison inhale the eucalyptus, because it is known to help with stuffiness and to open airways. I also sprinkled some on the neck of his T-shirt to inhale as we drove to the hotel. Once we got to our room, I put the eucalyptus oil in the vaporizer I'd bought and added water. That misted the room with the eucalyptus smell. Thankfully, these things worked.

I tell this story because it's a good example of how important it is to be prepared when you travel with kids, especially those who have health conditions. It's also an example of how I continue to learn new things along the way. For example, I'd never thought to make eucalyptus a regular part of my travel kit. I had been using it at home, but had never thought to pack it. But after the Miami experience, I won't go anywhere without it.

Our family often travels within and outside the United States, both for my husband's business and for vacations, and we've been doing so since our kids were six weeks old. There are also plenty of times when my husband is working and the kids have time off from school, so I travel with our two children by myself. I have always loved travel, and feel that I was somewhat of a gypsy in my life before having kids. But you don't have to stop traveling and it doesn't have to be much more difficult just because you have kids. The biggest thing I've learned from years of travel with my children is that if you're not prepared, it can cause frustration, stress, and anxiety. Being ready for anything alleviates that. We have no crystal ball, so we don't know what tomorrow will hold. Being organized and on top of things can help. Here are some of the important things that help make traveling with kids easier, safer, and more fun.

Avoid Unexpected Emotions

Because of my husband's unusual schedule, our vacations can change at a moment's notice, so I try not to tell my kids about a trip too far in advance. I'd rather surprise them with an unexpected vacation than disappoint them by canceling one they knew about. This is why I wait until the morning of a trip to tell them about it. Another reason I wait is that the excitement of an upcoming trip may make it hard for them to sleep or cause them to ask a million questions. So we avoid the anticipation and possible disappointment. You just never know when weather, a change of plans, or something else will cancel your trip.

Keep It Simple Through Security

- **Prep for the Security Line.** If you're traveling by plane, leave yourself extra time to go through security. And if you're traveling with children, be prepared to possibly have to remove their shoes and jackets and take their electronics out of their bags. I always have my children go through security in front of me, and I keep all the electronic items (like an iPod, iPad, iTouch, laptop, and portable DVD players) in my bag. This way I'm the only one who needs to pull things out and my kids aren't digging through their backpacks or bags.

- **Travel Light.** I also try to travel light. Now that they're older, I also make sure my kids can carry most of their own stuff. When they were younger, my rule was that if I was unable to carry it comfortably, I didn't bring it. I'd remind myself that this was not a rest-of-my-life trip, so I didn't need to bring everything we owned.

- **Purchase Your Beverages After Security.** Since you can't bring your own bottled water or other beverages through security, I make sure to buy water once we are close to the gate. Again, you can get beverages on the plane, but they won't serve these until you're at a certain altitude and it's safe to do so. What happens if you get thirsty, need to take a vitamin/medication, or need to clear your throat before then? Be prepared. If we're traveling by car and are with someone who has a tendency to get car sick, I may also pack some ginger ale (and a big enough plastic bag in case they need to throw up. This has happened to us twice).

- **"Gate-check" the Stroller.** When Arianna and Addison were younger, I'd take the stroller with me all the way to the gate and then "gate-check" it. This is when you wheel the stroller all the way to the plane's door. Then you leave it in a specific spot, where someone from the airline picks it up, stores it, and has it waiting for you right outside the airplane's door when you arrive at your destination. It makes life much easier, and you can use the stroller to help you carry things within the airport before boarding. (Just be careful not to load up the handlebars or the stroller can tip over backward. This can be very dangerous if your child is in the stroller; instead stash things under the stroller seat.) If you have two young kids, in my experience a double stroller and the airport just don't go well together. Instead, I got one of those skateboard-type adapters to put on the back of the stroller so Arianna could ride while Addison sat. And when she didn't want to ride, I used that platform for baggage.

Have Snacks on Hand (Lots of Them)

Because my kids have allergies and I prefer to give them real food over air-plane food, I'm used to carrying our own food. And when we travel, I make sure we have *a lot of it*. Airports don't always have things my kids can eat or things we want to eat, not to mention that the food they do have is expensive. I also know not to count on the airlines to serve anything. These days, the amount and kind of food they offer varies so much, not only from one airline to another, but from one flight to the next. So even if there is something we can eat on our outgoing flight, they don't always serve that same food on our flight home. Also, whether your child has food allergies or not, an air-line can't serve any food or drinks until the plane has push backed from the gate, taken off, and reached a certain altitude. If your kids get hungry before that happens—and mine tend to—you're in trouble if you don't have your own snacks. Plus, I've been in the situation where we're stuck on the runway because of a delay and have had to wait an additional forty-five minutes or longer for food service. When I carry my own food on board, and plenty of it, I'm ready for any delay, and I don't have the added stress of having cranky kids on my hands. (*We* cause the stress, not our kids. We blame them for their behavior, but it's really caused by our unpreparedness.) The bottom line is that when kids are cranky and hungry, traveling can be frustrating for all of you. When they're content and happy, you're content and happy, and travel-ing can actually be fun.

Some of my favorite travel snacks are turkey sandwiches, applesauce, pretzels, muffins, chips, and fruit snacks. (Because they are chewy, fruit snacks help my kids' ears during takeoff and landing. And I try to bring the ones with decent ingredients.)

As I mentioned in chapter 1, I sometimes bring foods such as applesauce and yogurt on the plane. Because these foods have a liquid consistency, they're not normally allowed through airport security, so I carry a signed and dated letter from our doctor explaining my children's food allergies and what foods we'll be carrying with us. This has been a huge help several times.

Choose Your Seats Strategically

When I travel with just my children (and not another adult), I purchase our seats in economy/coach to make it as cost-efficient as possible. I get three seats that are together and I sit in the middle so I can tend to the child on my left and the child on my right. This way there is no passing of items through the aisle or across the laps of strangers and no loud voices asking me questions such as, "Mommy, where is my game or my book? Will you please pass it to me?" Sitting in the middle, I can easily bend over and reach into that carry-on bag underneath the seat in front of me and dig around for whatever is needed. This appears to work for us and makes traveling a little less stressful. We are together, content, well-fed, and prepared! I also try not to get the bulkhead seats, which means there are no seats in front of you, so nowhere to put your bag.

Bring On the Entertainment

On long trips, or in case of delays, kids can get bored and restless, and once again, a cranky child can make traveling unpleasant—make that very unpleasant—for you and everyone around you. When my kids were younger, we often traveled back and forth between Atlanta and New York. For some reason, the flight to Atlanta was always delayed. The first few times, I didn't have enough things with me to entertain my kids, or I didn't have snacks on hand because I thought we'd be on time. Let's just say it was not an easy situation. I'd dig in my purse to see what I could use as entertainment for a toddler while also nursing an infant. Sometimes it was a flashlight on a keychain, which I shined on the back of the seat in front of me. Each trip teaches you what to add the next time, and I certainly learned my lesson from those flights: never leave home without snacks and some type of entertainment, both for the flight and once you reach your destination.

- **Paper and washable markers.** I don't care how old your child is, markers and a pad of paper can provide lots of entertainment. The children can draw, play games such as Hangman and Tic Tac Toe, trace their hands, or write a story. Yes, we live in a high-tech world, but good old-fashioned pen and paper can really keep kids busy. Simply toss a pad or a few sheets of paper in a plastic bag with markers, crayons, or pencils and you're set. If your kids are young, stickers can also be fun to add to the mix.

- **A device for watching movies.** This can be anything from a portable DVD player, a laptop, iPod, or iPad. Just make sure that if it's a DVD player you remember to pack some DVDs. (It may sound obvious, but I have forgotten DVDs on occasion!) Or if you download movies, make sure they're actually on the device and ready to go. Pack headphones so that you don't disturb other travelers with the sound of your child's movie. (The headphones they hand out or sell on planes don't always fit a child's head or your personal technology device, because the plugs can be different.) Even if you're not a fan of your child using electronics, consider making an exception, as it may save you in the case of a major delay or meltdown (your child's or your own). And don't forget to charge your devices before leaving home and to pack those chargers for later!

- **A toy or two.** There's no need to pack your child's entire room or fill a suitcase with toys. Just bring a few age-appropriate things that will keep him entertained. And if possible, don't ask your child what he wants to bring. When I did that once, Addison grabbed a huge box of superhero toys (his giant Buzz Lightyear and an entire box of *Toy Story* characters). Sometimes it's good to bring toys that your children haven't seen in a while; this way they get excited. (If they grow tired of the toy again, instead of packing it to bring back home, you can always donate it to someone in the place you're visiting or leave it in the hotel room with a note for the housekeeper to keep the item or donate it.)

- **Books.** Just make sure they're paperback, travel-size books so you don't make your luggage heavier than it needs to be. Small activity books are also great for kids and are available for all ages, from simple coloring and connect-the-dot books to maze and crossword puzzle books for older kids. School-like workbooks with math and writing exercises are great, too, and make your trip a bit educational. If there's a book your child insists you read each night, you don't have to lug it with you. Just record it and play it during your trip. (This is also great to do if you have to go away without your child, so she can hear your voice while you're gone.)

- **Games.** Travel-size versions of your family's favorite games and decks of cards—Go Fish, Old Maid, and Uno—are easy to stash even in the smallest carry-on, and provide hours of fun. Our deck of Uno goes with us everywhere. I just toss it in a resealable plastic bag and throw it in my purse. When my kids were learning to read and do basic math, I brought flashcards.

- **Old-fashioned games.** There were plenty of times when my kids were babies that they were happily entertained with a game of Peek-aboo, Patty-Cake, or This Little Piggy Went to Market. You can also show them pictures stored in your phone and play Guess Who That Is.

- **A favorite blanket or stuffed animal.** If there's a blanket or stuffed animal your child *must* have in order to nap, fall asleep, or just feel comforted, bring it. Especially if you're going somewhere unfamiliar and you think your child will need this item to feel safe and comfortable. (But keep your eye on it so you don't forget to bring it back home.)

Stock Up on Baby Supplies

For such little human beings, babies seem to need an awful lot of supplies. Still, when my kids were babies, I tried to bring only the bare essentials, such as diapers, wipes, breast pads, and formula. I'd stash the extra, unused diapers in a resealable plastic bag and use that as my garbage when I needed a place for the dirty diaper. I also brought along extra resealable plastic bags, inside a resealable plastic bag, and still do this today. These bags are good for everything, from storing wet swimsuits and soiled undies, to carrying snacks, to serving as garbage bags, or to use if someone needs to throw up.

Bring Extra Clothes

I used to think this was a good tip for my kids only when they were babies and they had accidents. But it's still relevant even now that they're older, because you never know when turbulence or carelessness will cause a drink to spill or when a case of sudden diarrhea will occur. If you don't have extra clothes, your child will be cold and uncomfortable, and you'll hear about it. With extra clothes, you can get him changed and comfy fast. And this isn't just a tip for your kids. I stash a set of extra clothes for myself in my carry-on bag.

I also make sure we have sweatshirts and/or jackets, because even if the outside temperature is warm, the plane and airport are always freezing, thanks to air-conditioning. It's better to layer up and take things off than to be cold (or worse, to have to buy a high-priced sweatshirt at the airport because your kids are shivering). If we're coming from somewhere cold and are dressed in winter garb but are going to a warm destination, the kids put T-shirts or tank tops under their sweaters, so they can peel off the layers when we arrive. On the other extreme, if we leave somewhere warm in short sleeves and shorts, I pack long-sleeve shirts and sweatshirts they can slip on during the plane ride. There are also coats and hats in our carry-ons they can wear when we arrive.

Make Your Own Travel Kit

Whether we go away for one night or two weeks, and whether we travel across town or out of the country, I don't leave home without a travel kit I've put together. It contains essential items that I always have in case my kids get sick or hurt. You can never know. Your children can be healthy when you leave for vacation, but pick up something or get hurt while you're away. If you have nothing with you, you'll be stressed and frazzled as you scramble for help.

- **A thermometer.** When we were in the Caribbean when Arianna was six months old, she woke up one day with diarrhea and felt warm. I called our pediatrician, whose first question was "Does she have a fever?" I have no idea why I'd brought a thermometer with me, but I'm glad I had, and have traveled with one ever since. A fever is a sign of something, so no matter which doctor you call or hospital you take your child to, body temperature is important and necessary information.

- **Fever reducers.** If you use them, take them with you. I carry both a traditional fever reducer, such as Motrin, along with a homeopathic version. Sometimes you can get the main brands of fever reducers abroad and sometimes you can't. Stores may not always be open when you need them, and if you're in an airport or a hotel gift shop, the fever reducers they have may be expensive or unfamiliar.

- **Doctors' phone numbers.** These are stored in my cell phone, but I still have them written on a piece of paper, which I keep with our medical/toiletry kit just in case I'm not near my phone or if a babysitter is watching the kids.

- **Kids' medical bracelets.** Because of our allergies, I got my children medical bracelets to wear when we travel. This is especially important if I put them in a kids' club or drop them at a friend's house. In those situations, I may tell one caregiver that my children have allergies, but she might forget to pass this information on to the other caregivers. (My children also wear these bracelets during the first few weeks of school, until their teachers are familiar with which allergies they have, and for school field trips, because parent chaperones may not know my kids.) You can get all sorts of cute, fashionable medical bracelets that kids will actually want to wear.

- **My medical bracelet.** I also wear a medical bracelet when we travel. This is really important if I'm the only adult traveling with my children. My kids know what I'm allergic to, but in an emergency situation they may not remember.

- **An albuterol inhaler.** Even though we rarely use it, there are times, such as that incident at the Miami airport, when it was needed. I want to be prepared and responsible just in case.

- **Benadryl and EpiPens.** Again, I'm not big on medicine, but if one of us has an allergic reaction I want to be ready. Be sure to include the instructions for using the EpiPen, in case a flight attendant or other stranger must use it on you or your kids. And make sure none of your medication has expired.

- **Health insurance cards.** If you have to see a doctor when you're out of town, they will not have this information on file the way your regular doctor will, so bring it with you.

- **Birth medical cards.** These are cards my pediatrician gave us when my kids were born and which she updates with their height, weight, and vaccination information at each well visit. (Even if you choose not to vaccinate, you'll still want to have this information updated and on hand.) I photocopy the cards, leave the originals at home, and take the copies with me. This way, in the event of a medical emergency, I'll know which shots my children have already had. After all, you don't want anyone to administer a shot your child doesn't need, and if your child hasn't received a specific shot and it's an emergency, the doctor needs to know that, too.

- **Homeopathic remedies.** Be sure to bring along products such as tea tree cream, which is an antiseptic that's good for cleaning cuts; eucalyptus, which is good for inhaling and opening air passages, and treating coughs and stuffed noses; arnica, which is good for bruises and soreness; and calendula ointment, for cuts, burns, chapping, and scrapes.

- **A homeopathic kit.** I ordered this kit online. It comes with a hundred homeopathic remedies, tiny tubes of pellets you can take for a variety of ailments. It has a remedy for anything you experience—from food poisoning to bee stings to ear infections—and it lasts for years. It also includes a pamphlet with a breakdown of what each homeopathic remedy can be used for. (The one I like is from Washington Homeopathic Products.)

- **Hot/cold water bottle.** This rubber vessel lies flat when it's empty, so it doesn't take up too much space in your luggage. It's great for filling with ice or hot water to soothe sore and pulled muscles and bumps and bruises.

- **Acupressure point wrist bands.** These look like cute bracelets, but have a little plastic nub that presses on a specific pressure point on the wrist to alleviate motion sickness. I have these in both adult and kid sizes, in case anyone experiences motion sickness. They're good for planes, cars, boat rides, trains—anything motion related.

- **Resealable plastic bags.** These have a million uses, and one of them is as a cold water bottle: just fill it with ice cubes. Use them if someone gets car sick, or if your toddler needs to go to the bathroom but there's no restroom in sight. (Yes, you can use a resealable plastic bag for urine. After all, it's probably safer for your child to stay in the car than to get out on a dark road to pee.)

- **Parental consent letter.** Whenever I travel without my husband, especially out of the country, I make sure to bring a signed letter from him with his permission in writing that he is aware that I am taking my kids away on my own. Airport, airline, and immigration officials may not ask for it, but sometimes they will. I like to be prepared just in case.

If you travel often, I'd suggest having your travel kit packed at all times. I never unpack mine; I just restock it if I've used up any items and check to make sure those with expiration dates, such as medications, ointments, and creams, aren't too old.

Choose Your Hotel Carefully

Because of my children's allergies, I try to stay at hotels where they have a twenty-four-hour concierge. This way they can assist me if my kids need medical attention; they're generally available all day and all night. If the hotel doesn't have a concierge, find out where the nearest hospital is located. You never know if and when you'll need it. (In my experience, it's usually in the middle of the night when someone gets sick.)

Make Your Trip Allergy-Proof

I mentioned this in chapter 1, but I think it bears repeating. If you're traveling to a place where you don't speak the language, make sure you can explain your kids' allergies in that language. Try to find a local who speaks your language—either before you go away or at the hotel. Tell him what your children are allergic to and ask him how to say it in his language. Ask him to write the word down so that later, at a hospital or doctor's office, if you're mis-understood, you can show the doctor the written word. I also bring a transla-tion book. There are apps for foreign languages for cell phones, but you don't want to depend on them, because you may not get service or your phone's battery may be dead. (For more information, see chapter 1.)

ANSWERS FROM ERICA'S EXPERT

Sara Keagle has been a flight attendant for a major U.S. airline for the past eighteen years and has spent the last twenty in the travel industry. As a result, she has been in a position to observe many, many families traveling. This, coupled with her passion for parenting, makes her an invaluable resource for family travel tips and ideas. Through her website The Flying Pinto (the flyingpinto.com) she shares her experiences and offers a glimpse behind the galley curtain. She has also created and cohosts a popular podcast, The Crew Lounge, which offers listeners a unique look at the life and career of a flight attendant. Sara has also freelanced for *The Wall Street Journal*'s *Speak Easy* blog and serves as a resource for various national media outlets, including *USA Today*, *The Wall Street Journal*, MSNBC, *The New York Times*, *Budget Travel*, *Trip Base*, and *The Washington Post*. She is the mother of a four-year-old girl.

Travel Tips

What are the top five things to bring in your carry-on bag for your baby?
1. **Diapers and wipes.** My rule of thumb is one diaper for every hour of my journey plus five. Delays from mechanicals or weather happen fre-quently enough, and I have seen too many parents run out of diapers while stuck on a plane. Not fun for anyone! If you do find yourself in this situation, look for other people traveling with babies.
2. **Food supply.** If you're breast-feeding, great; if not, bring enough for-mula. Again, enough for the journey plus a little extra. Always check

the Transportation Security Administration (TSA) website, TSA.gov, for updated regulations, but formula, milk, and breast milk are currently allowed in quantities larger than 3.4 ounces. It is also a great idea to plan on feeding your baby during takeoff and descent. If their ears bother them, this will help. The noise during takeoff always put my baby to sleep.

3. **Resealable plastic bags.** These are great for dirty diapers and/or soiled clothing. A flight attendant won't take a used diaper from you, even if she is collecting trash. It is not because she is being rude. Flight attendants handle food, and our trash is stored in the galley (the kitchen), and health codes stipulate that dirty diapers must be disposed of in the lavatories by the passenger.

4. **Extra clothes.** Bring extras for the baby, an extra shirt for Mom or Dad, and a small blanket or two.

5. **Ear plugs.** I pack enough for all my neighbors on the plane, just in case things get out of control. It allows me to stress less knowing I have them.

What are the top five things to bring in your carry-on bag for your toddlers or older children?

1. **Snacks.** Think healthy snacks. You may think sweets would be a nice treat for the plane, but you're better off offering that treat after you've made it to your destination. You need your kids' blood sugar levels to stay steady. Nuts, granola bars, and fruit are all great snacks. For longer flights, I pack plain pasta (great finger food) and frozen mixed vegetables (they thaw out in time to eat). Think about what your kids enjoy that's on the healthy side and not too messy.

2. **Disposable place mats and wipes.** You can buy these at most supermarkets, and they are a must. If you put one on the tray table after takeoff, your kids can eat and play germ-free. Airplane cleaners have an average of seven minutes to clean in between flights, so tray tables usually get cleaned only once a day.

3. **Activities.** Bring things your child enjoys. DVD players, books, sticker books, paper dolls, triangle crayons (so they don't roll), and erasable activity books are a few good ideas.

4. **Empty water bottles.** These can include Sigg and Klean Kanteen bottles. Always fill your water bottles at the water bubbler once through security. It saves time (that you may not have) and money (on plastic bottles).

5. **CARES (Child Aviation Restraint System).** This is a harness-type child aviation safety restraint certified by the Federal Aviation Administration (FAA). It is for children twenty-two to forty-four pounds. You simply place it around the airplane seat and adjust the straps to fit your child. It then loops through the regular seat belt, and your child is harnessed in. It is also very lightweight (one pound) and packs easily into your carry-on. A CARES will retail for about eighty dollars, so it is pricey, but worth it if you travel a lot. A great idea is to buy one with a neighbor or relative and split the cost. Chances are you won't be traveling at the same time.

Is there a best age/age range to start traveling with children?

If you have the opportunity I say the sooner the better. I would check with your health care provider for the best time to start. My daughter has been on a plane almost every other month since she was an infant. She loves to fly and is also one of the best passengers I know, adult or child!

Do you have to buy a baby a plane ticket? If so, is it offered at a discounted price?

No, you are not required to buy a plane ticket for children under the age of two. However, the absolute safest way to travel with an infant by plane is in a rear-facing car seat (one that is FAA approved), just as in your car. The airlines generally do not offer discounted seats for children. If you're traveling internationally, be prepared to pay a surcharge of around 10 percent of the fare plus any international taxes for a child who doesn't have a seat and will be sitting on your lap (called "lap children"). Check with your airline when booking your tickets.

What's the safest way to travel with a toddler by plane?

A car seat or a CARES (Child Aviation Restraint System). I love CARES because it is easy to pack, carry, and set up. I also love that my child doesn't end up kicking the seat in front of her, as she would in a car seat. I check the car seat curbside and have never had a problem with it arriving damaged. It makes going through security so much easier, too.

Do you need to use a car seat on a plane, and for what age? Or is it safe to hold a baby on your lap?

You don't need the car seat, but I recommend you use one until your child weighs twenty-two pounds. (You can buy a strap that allows you to attach the car seat to your rollerboard). After twenty-two pounds, you can switch to a CARES. In the event of a crash or in turbulence, it is not safe to hold your infant, so you're taking a calculated risk when doing so.

Is there anything you recommend for your children's ears as you take off and land?

I recommend anything that causes them to suck, whether it is breast-feeding, a bottle, a pacifier, or gum for older kids. Drinking plenty of water is also important, because the cabin's dry air can thicken nasal mucus, making it more likely that the Eustachian tubes (which equalize pressure in the ears) will become clogged. If your child has known problems with her ears or has a cold, I recommend giving her ibuprofen about a half hour before takeoff and, if the flight is longer than the next recommended dose, again during landing.

Which is the best seat to buy if traveling on a plane with kids—i.e., is it the back of the plane, middle, or front? Aisle or window? Bulkhead?

The back of the plane or closest to the lavatories is a good spot for families, but if you have an infant, some planes have bassinets that attach to the bulkhead row for the cruise portion of flight. (Check with the airline when booking.) I also find that kids love to look out the window!

What if your child has an allergy to a certain food or snack being served on the plane (such as nuts). What do you do in that case?

If your child has a known allergy, discuss it with the airline representative when booking your ticket. Even if the airline agrees not to serve the food your child is allergic to, there could be passengers on board with that food.

I would let the gate agents and the flight attendants know about your child's allergy so that they are able to make an announcement. Keep in mind that not all airlines will accommodate this request, so make sure you have any meds you need in your carry-on and not in your checked baggage.

Is it possible to call ahead about food on an upcoming flight?

You can call or look online to see what food offerings are available on your upcoming flight. Most domestic U.S. airlines do not serve free or special meals, but if you are flying internationally or on some foreign carriers, you can call or go online to place your special request.

When it comes to boarding a plane with children, what are the pros and cons to boarding before the other passengers?

There are definitely a couple of pros to boarding early. You are able to get settled without the passengers behind you waiting, and you get first dibs on the overhead space. I like to get out some activities and anything else I might need before the seat belt sign is released. The con is that anytime a child is confined for a long time, it is tricky, and the longer he's confined, the worse it gets. The best of both worlds is if you are traveling with two adults. Have one adult hang out with the kids in the boarding area, hopefully getting out any last-minute energy until final call, while the other adult (designated pack mule) preboards with all the stuff.

What's the best way to change a baby's diaper on an airplane?

Most airplanes now have changing tables in the lavatories. If you find it absolutely necessary to change your child at your seat, do not do it on the tray table. Remember, the tray tables are not cleaned in between flights.

If you're traveling alone with a child and have to go to the bathroom, what can you do? It is it okay to ask a flight attendant to watch your child?

What I do is look for another mom sitting close to me. I will ask her to watch over my daughter if she is asleep. If she is awake, she comes with me. You can ask the flight attendant, but some airlines have policies in place that do not allow flight attendants to hold babies.

What's the best way to keep kids busy when traveling by any means (plane, car, train)?

It really depends on your kids. Whatever quiet activities they enjoy at home will be best. Some kids enjoy movies while other kids like journaling, coloring, or writing in activity books.

If you aren't prepared with toys and games, what do you suggest for keeping kids entertained?

Storytelling or creative games such as I Spy. I found a great memory game from a deck of cards called Fifty-Two Things to Do on a Plane. One person starts out saying, "I packed my suitcase with (blank)"; then the next person says, "I packed my suitcase with (the item the first person mentioned and a new item)." You continue, with everyone adding an item and repeating all the items that have been listed thus far and do so until someone forgets one item from the list. You can also ask a neighbor for a pen and play Tic Tac Toe and/or Hangman using space you can find in the airplane catalog for paper.

What if you don't have food with you and your child is thirsty or hungry before the flight attendants are allowed to serve food?

Never leave home without snacks. But if you do, buy some snacks at the airport. If you don't have time and you find yourself stuck, explain your situation to the flight attendant. But keep in mind that flight attendants may not have any food to offer. Again, I would look for a mom. I've often helped out moms who didn't have snacks for their kids by finding a mom with snacks.

How do you make relations with other passengers better when you've got a screaming child on a plane?

Ear plugs. Bring a package of them in your carry-on. It will break the ice; plus it's hard to be mad at someone who's making an effort. Still, keep in mind that some people are going to be mean and/or angry no matter what you do to remedy the situation. There will also be people who think no matter what you are doing it is wrong. Hand out the ear plugs, and then do what is best for your child. Babies cry. Toddlers have tantrums, especially under stress, so that means taking care of yourself, too. Be prepared for travel, pack a full day in advance, do the best you can to calm and relax your child, and once you have exhausted all avenues, relax, knowing that your baby or toddler will wear himself out eventually and probably fall asleep for the rest of the flight.

What's the best way to prepare a toddler or older child for traveling?

Give yourself oodles of time. Your kids feed off your emotions: if you're stressed, they will be stressed. Have enough time to get on their level and let them know what is ahead of them. Involve them in the planning as much as possible. If your kids are small, read books to them about flying ahead of time, start pointing out airplanes in the sky, and get them excited about the trip. You can involve older kids more by having them help pack, making a checklist, etc. If you are going someplace new, go to the library and read about your destination. Also, let your kids know ahead of time that they will need to wear their seat belt for the whole trip. This may help, if they have that expectation.

What are your tips for going through airport security with children?

If you have a baby, wear a sling. It leaves your hands free, and most TSA agents won't make you take it off. Again, check with TSA.gov for updated information. Also, remember that security lines can be long, especially if you are traveling during peak times. Kids can get antsy there, too, so have activities in mind, such as I Spy. Have your children wear slip-on shoes and belt-free clothing.

From a flight attendant's perspective, what are some of the most annoying things parents do while traveling with their kids, and solutions?

Most of the annoying things parents do are from lack of experience. Most parents aren't ever in such tight quarters with their kids, except maybe the car, and the kids are buckled in the whole time. Some of the more troublesome things parents do is let their kids run wild, ring the call light, and (one of my personal pet peeves) make a huge mess and leave it. How can you remedy these situations? By being prepared with activities and not giving kids too much sugar before or during the flight. If you find or think you will have a lot of trash, ask the flight attendant for a trash bag to keep at your seat. As far as loud games and toys go, most airlines have a rule that you need to use headphones on all electronics with sound. There are some amazing headphones specially made for children, with volume control (so kids can't blast their eardrums). They are adult quality and cost about twenty dollars.

If you have the option, which time of day is the best time to travel with kids (by any means)?

The earlier the better. Everyone will be fresh, and you'll have a better chance of flights leaving on time in the morning. There are far fewer delays in the morning. Flights have a tendency to get backed up as the day progresses.

If your child is sick and you've already bought your ticket, do you cancel your ticket or stick with it so as not to waste the money?

This really depends on you and your child. What does your child have? If it is a mild cold, I would give him ibuprofen before the flight and go. If he's running a fever, I would cancel. Remember, you will be exposed to many germs while traveling. I would put my child's health ahead of losing money.

As a travel insider, is there anything you can tell us about hygiene on the plane?

Yes. You will be exposed to hundreds of people's germs just by touching the lavatory door handle. The airplane cleaners have a very small window of time to clean the airplanes, and they don't clean the door handles. That means if you are on an 8:00 p.m. flight and that aircraft flew five or six flights that day and there were 140 or so people on each flight—well, you can do the math! These are germs from all over the world. I was sick more in my first year of being a flight attendant than at any other time in my life. Remember, too, that when most people fly they are stressed. Add that to how tiring it is to fly and... voilà! You have a recipe for getting sick. So what can you do? Wash your hands, don't touch your face, and make sure you have antibacterial wipes with you. When I am home I just use soap, but on the road I use antibacterial products.

When traveling with school-age children, do you suggest they carry their own bags or do you carry them?

Until you know that your child is capable of being responsible for her own bag the whole time, pack what I call the "family suitcase." It's really going to depend on the age of your child and how far and/or long your journey is. If your small child has her own suitcase (which is tempting; they're very cute), guess who will be lugging it? Yes, you! I can pack my clothes and enough clothes for two children in my twenty-inch rollerboard. I use a space-saver bag, which, after you unpack at your destination, becomes your laundry bag. When you are ready to pack for your trip home, just push on the bag to get the air out—no vacuum cleaner needed.

How many bags do you suggest traveling with?

I recommend as few bags as possible. One twenty- to twenty-two-inch carry-on per adult, a tote for each adult, and a cooler for the snacks. If your kids really want to carry something, I would get them a *very* lightweight backpack and put a very light stuffed animal or something else lightweight in it. Make sure it'll fit in your bag if needed.

Any other tips for traveling with kids?

Yes.

- If you are by yourself and have several children, ask for help when checking in. People think to ask for an electric cart after a flight, but you can ask for one to get to your gate, too.
- Other great products when flying with kids are solid shampoos and bath products. You won't have to worry about your liquids exploding, and they make going through security a breeze.
- Bring enough baby supplies for your travel day and order the rest through diapers.com or a similar service so the supplies are at your destination when you arrive. You'll save a ton of precious luggage space and won't have to run to the store after a long travel day because you've forgotten something.
- Once we had children, we started renting houses through websites that help you find rental homes (homeaway.com or VRBO.com), instead of booking hotel rooms. The cost is comparable and you have use of a kitchen, which helps you save a lot of money.
- Remember that with more kids come more carry-ons than you are allowed (one per person plus a purse, diaper bag, cooler, etc.—so

essentially two per person, one large, one small). Don't waste that on small children's suitcases. Instead add a soft-sided cooler and pack it with enough snacks for the day. There are coolers that will attach and sit right on top of your rollerboard.

- Overall, remember to enjoy the journey. I see flying as a way to spend quality time with my family without interruption from the day's usual activities. I skip the electronics and play with my child.

- Ask the flight attendant when you get on the plane if your children can say hi to the pilots. Most pilots love to show the flight deck to kids. Remember to give yourself lots of time and to see the day through your kids' eyes. It can be pretty magical.

PART II

AN EMOTIONALLY THRIVING CHILD

Chapter 8

Raising Kids with Respect, Responsibilities, and Discipline

I was confronted with the challenge of raising three daughters as a single parent. The job doesn't come with a manual, but I tackled it head-on and gave it my best shot. I realized that in order to be successful at my duty, I needed to be heard and understood. So I developed a voice of authority that gained respect and obedience. Through my leadership, I created an orderly home and guidance. In waves I strived to invest good character in them. My children took heed to my direction and understood that a certain stare or head bopping could mean trouble.

—Margie Sherard, mother of three girls

One day when my daughter was three years old, we made a batch of cupcakes. After mixing and baking, we decorated the cupcakes with pink frosting, and then Arianna excitedly sprinkled edible pastel hearts on top. She loved those cupcakes. She was so excited about them. We each ate a delicious cupcake and then arranged the rest on a pretty plate and set them aside for the next day. It was a lovely moment shared between the two of us.

But that night, while I was putting Arianna to bed, she got sassy with me. I can't remember exactly what she did, but she gave me some sort of attitude that was inappropriate. (Though my daughter skipped what some call "the terrible twos," we did experience the "sassy threes.") So I gave her a warning: "If you do that again," I said firmly, "those cupcakes are going in the garbage." A few minutes later, she did whatever I had warned her not to do. She was testing me. The threat about tossing the cupcakes in the garbage had slipped out of my mouth a bit unexpectedly. *Oh my gosh*, I thought. *We're going to throw away those delicious cupcakes!* I knew at this point that I wanted to take back that threat, but I also knew I had to use this moment as a learning experience for us both. She needed to learn that Mommy means what she says, and I needed to learn to follow through. So I didn't back down. I didn't offer her twelve more chances. I followed through.

I took Arianna out of her bed (I know it sounds a little *Mommy Dearest*, but it wasn't that bad!) and I walked toward the kitchen. She trailed behind me crying hard and loud, "No, Mommy. Not my cupcakes. No." I stayed focused. I walked into the kitchen and picked up the plate of cupcakes. But I wasn't going to throw them in the kitchen garbage, where we would be able to see them. Oh no. I wanted her to know that I was serious and that those cupcakes were gone for good, so I walked into the hallway of our apartment building and opened the door to the incinerator. She had to witness me throwing her pretty cupcakes down that long, dark chute. She screamed and cried. It hurt to hear her and see her like this, but I knew this was a necessary experience. She had a tantrum. It wasn't pretty, but I knew if I didn't stand firm and do what I had said I would and make my point, my words would appear to be meaning-less to her in the future. And she might not take me seriously when it came to discipline and consequences for certain unacceptable behavior.

The other thing that worked was giving her something I call "the eye": a look from me that told her I meant business. I didn't have to say a word. All I had to do was glance over at her with "the eye" and she'd behave (well, most of the time). This worked beautifully until she was about five years old. Unfor-tunately, "the eye" didn't work for Addison. (Time-outs worked better for him when he was young.) Instead, it only made him cry. It bothered him in a different way, which taught me that just because you have two children it doesn't mean they will respond to the same type of discipline.

Today, what I do in place of giving them "the eye" is tell them I will count to five and when I get to five I will follow through with whatever consequence I warned them about. For example, say Addison is playing his video game and I call him to the dinner table. If I have to call him more than two times and he still has not budged from his game, I say, "I am about to start counting and if I get to five, you can't play any more games for the rest of the day. I am counting now. One, two..." Usually by three, he has joined us at the table to eat. I do this for both my children. It has really worked for me and has been my saving grace after "the eye" stopped working.

Tough love is not easy. It hurts to discipline, but it also hurts to live with unruly kids. But if you tiptoe around them when they're toddlers because you don't want them to have tantrums, you have to be prepared to pay when they're thirteen, fourteen, or fifteen years old. I don't say "yes" to everything when they're young, because I don't want to raise kids who can't be told "no" when they're older. Saying "yes" all the time is a good way to lose control of your kids. I often wonder why we moms and dads are so afraid of tantrums anyway. A tantrum is often the only way our children know how to express emotions. It is how they learn to cope with feelings that are often rushing in at rapid speed.

Every child is unique and every child reacts differently to certain types of discipline. I'm simply sharing things from my home, my experience, and my children. You have to know what works for you and your kids, but one thing's for sure: discipline is crucial for happy, well-behaved children (not to mention sane moms). Keeping them healthy is critical. But it's also important to make sure your children thrive emotionally, which is what we'll focus on in the second half of this book.

Follow Through on Your Warnings

This is one of my keys to disciplining my kids. Recently, I noticed that my kids were fighting more than usual, and I was tired of it. I understand that they're two years apart, share a room, and can get on each other's nerves, but this constant bickering over the silliest things was getting to me. So I took away their computers and video games until spring break, which was about six weeks away. I also told them that they were not going to have any more playdates until they got along.

"You can't bring friends into our home if you can't work things out and be nice to each other," I told them.

Later that day Addison said, "Mommy, we decided that we're going to get along."

But they'd said that before. "I want to see action," I replied.

The point is that I have to look at what my children care about and then use that to help discipline them. For example, my son is really into his Wii, Xbox, his laptop, and pretty much anything that has to do with technology, so if I tell him that those items may be taken away, he seems to get the point. Though video games aren't that important to Arianna, she really cares about playdates. In my opinion, these things should be earned. They shouldn't just be handed to kids.

I need to be consistent with my discipline the same way that I need to be consistent with my love.

Make Manners Count

Manners are a big deal to me. Today's world is much different from when our great-grandparents, grandparents, or even we were growing up. But just because the world is flying by at the blink of the eye, and much of our communication is high tech, doesn't mean we can bypass having basic manners and teaching them to our children. It doesn't mean we should lose the ability to deal with other human beings. Think like Aretha Franklin when she sings R-E-S-P-E-C-T. We have to respect our children, and they have to respect us. And we have to teach them to respect others. That's partly why I have my kids share a room. I want them to learn to respect another person's space and things.

My kids have been taught to look everyone in the eye, from the dog groomer to their piano teacher, to me and their father. When my children go on a playdate, I want them to greet the other child's parent or caregiver before heading to their friend's room. And when the playdate is over, I want them to thank the adult and say good-bye. That's what I did when I was a kid. So many children don't even acknowledge the adults in the room anymore. Not even with a simple "hello." (What makes me nuts is when the adult standing next to that child doesn't notice this or remind the child to say hello.) This is something we need to teach our children, and we're the only ones who can do it. I remember hearing one mom ask her son's preschool teacher, "Can you please teach Aidan how to say 'please' and 'thank you' at home?" Isn't that *our* job as mothers and fathers? This is not what a teacher is supposed to do. We, the parents, are *the* constant teachers in our kids' lives. Schoolteachers are there to feed our children's minds and foster their education. They can support our children in a loving, challenging way while they're at school and in their care. They can reinforce good behavior. But teaching manners is our job. And it's one I take seriously.

I was recently on a plane with my children, and after the flight a woman came up to me and said, "Your children are so well behaved." I thanked her, but what I was really thinking was, *What are you used to seeing? How are they supposed to behave?* This goes along with another rule of mine, which is that if you don't have what I call "home training," then you're not going to have restaurant training. By this I mean that when we're at home, I teach my kids how to act when we're out in the world. My kids also write thank-you notes for gifts; in my experience few kids seem to do that these days. It's something so basic, yet so important. After all, how hard is it to write a brief thank-you note or e-mail to acknowledge a gift and show your appreciation for someone else?

Another thing I've had to teach my kids is to say "excuse me" when they need to ask me something and I'm on the phone or talking to another adult. Sometimes they're good, but there are plenty of times when I have to say, "Do you see two adults speaking?" or "If you see Mommy speaking to another adult you have to say, 'Excuse me, Mommy.' " I also bring it to their attention that just because they say, "Excuse me," it doesn't mean I'll stop my conversation and drop everything for them right away.

Many aspects of discipline and manners are a work in progress. It's not like potty training, where once your kids figure out how to do it, they're done. There are certain things you have to teach continually. Sometimes I feel like a broken record and get sick of hearing myself reminding my kids to do things, but eventually it sinks in.

Give Children Responsibilities

In our home, my children have chores and responsibilities. If they don't do them, they don't get their allowance on Saturday. Their chores include making their own beds, setting the table, feeding the dog, keeping their room clean, bringing in the newspaper, and (sometimes) taking out the trash. I don't believe that kids should be rewarded for things they're supposed to do, so I never say, "If you get dressed, you'll get *x*, *y*, and *z*." I don't want them to do their chores only because they think they're going to be rewarded. I want them to do those things because it's what they're supposed to do. It's part of the responsibility of having your own bed and a dog, etc. When I give them their allowance, I make sure they know why. "This is not a reward," I tell them. "You worked for this."

Speaking of allowance and money, before we go into a store I'll tell my kids how much money they can spend. I establish this up front, so there's no negotiating or disagreeing if, once they get inside, they want something that's too expensive. This teaches my kids arithmetic, and it forces them to look at the price tags of items they want. I don't let them buy something every time we go into a store, but on the occasions I do, this is how I handle it. If they have their chore money with them, they can buy something with that.

Give Yourself a Chance to Cool Down

One recent morning, the school bus driver called to tell me that my kids were fighting on the bus and that it had been going on for a while. The bus driver! I was stunned. No one had ever had to call me about my kids' behavior.

I had the driver put the kids on the phone and I said to them, "You guys messed up big time! We'll talk when you get home."

When I picked them up from school that day I said, "Do you understand the seriousness of this? The bus driver actually had to call me while he was working, in the middle of his job, to tell me how my kids were acting."

I don't know why they were in this bickering stage, but obviously there was a problem: they had taken this beyond the bedroom and to the bus, and that's unacceptable. If the bus driver has to call, that is a call to arms for me. It means something requires attention or I need to handle something differently.

This situation taught me that it was good that I didn't react right away. I had a lot of time to cool down. I had from the morning to 3:00 p.m., which is pickup time, to think about how I was going to handle the situation. This was time in which I could decide not to yell or get upset, but to let them know I meant business and that their behavior was unacceptable. It worked.

Later that day, when I was talking to them about it, they were listening to me. They were glued. First, I let each of them tell me their side of the story. Then I told them, "You have to write fifty times, 'I will not pick on you, Arianna' and 'I will not pick on you, Addison.'" They also had to write, "I'm sorry for picking on you, Arianna" and "I'm sorry for picking on you, Addison." They had to turn all this in to me by Sunday at 10:00 a.m. at the latest. If they did not, they'd lose all their electronics until after spring break. When they completed this writing, I helped them tape it to their bedroom wall, so they would be able to see that they had said they wouldn't behave that way anymore. They also weren't allowed to watch TV, use the phone, or have any playdates over the weekend. And they had to apologize to the bus driver. At first I was going to have them simply write him a note of apology, but then I said, "Better yet, you are both to go up to him first thing Monday morning, look him straight in the eye, and apologize for your behavior." I thought this was harder to do than write a note and just hand it to him. I finished by telling them that if this behavior continued, we'd donate their electronics to a stranger. They knew I meant business, because I follow through.

One of their innocent responses was "Can we delete our personal information before donating them?"

I finished by making them sign a contract that listed all these punishments. I made them read it aloud and tell me that they understood it, because I didn't want them to say later, "Oh, I didn't know that."

Refraining from reacting immediately truly gave me good thinking time to digest what had happened and figure out what to do as a result of their actions. Rather than being angry, I was able to talk to them calmly but firmly. I didn't raise my voice. And they listened to me. "I took the school bus at one point during my school years and my mother never spoke to the school bus driver," I told them. "He never called our home." They got the point. It felt good to do it calmly and with some thought. I think a lot of times we react out of emotion and too quickly. It really helped me that I was notified early in the day and was forced to put off discussing it with them until they'd come home from school.

Ever since then, their relationship with each other has been so much better. They still bicker, but it's not every morning and after school each day.

Create a United Front

In my home, I'm the disciplinarian. When my husband disciplines Addison and Arianna, he says things like "If you do that again, I'll cut your arm off." Obviously, they know that's not going to happen, so they think they can get away with stuff with him. (And often they do.) There are times when my kids will try to take advantage of this. They will even call my husband at work to get him to override one of my decisions. I have to tell them that he is not my dad; he is my husband. I am the adult here in our home and I am responsible. When they bring him into it, they don't always tell the full story. Once when I took my kids' electronics away until spring break (which was a month away), I heard Arianna ask her father if she could use his iPhone. "What's wrong with your iPod?" he asked her, to which she replied, "Mommy took it away and she won't give it back." That wasn't the full story. She was going to get it back when spring break arrived—a little detail she conveniently left out.

Set the Tone

There's a saying, "Actions speak louder than words," and this is true with children. They are always watching us. They are our mirrors. That's why we need to respect them and those around us, because they're watching and listening to us more than we know. Consciously or not, we teach them their manners and the proper way to behave.

A few years ago my son pointed out that I was always checking e-mail on my BlackBerry in their presence. "No, I'm not," I said defensively. But once he raised my awareness, I realized that I returned calls and e-mails while with them. I realized that after school I picked them up, greeted them with a big kiss and hug, questioned them about their day, and then—boom, there I was checking e-mails. My kids busted me on this behavior and they were right. Their telling me this made me see that I was not devoting 100 percent of my time to them. They did not have my undivided attention.

Sometimes now what I do is leave my BlackBerry at home instead of bringing it with me to take them to and from school. It was hard in the beginning, because I had gotten so used to being glued to it and constantly in touch with others, but I had to remind myself that this was a moment I was getting to spend with my children. What's more important?

Teach Your Kids to Set the Tone for Their Friends

It's important that my kids teach their friends how to act in our home. I explain to them that how they behave will model how their friends behave. They have to show respect for our home and belongings. For example, I tell Addison that when his sister's not home, he has to speak up and tell his friends that they are not allowed to touch her belongings. Little boys and girls can be very inquisitive. Some may want to play with certain things and dissect them (and may accidentally break them), but I remind him that you need permission to play with or touch another's things.

My kids also now know that it's important to encourage their friends to clean up before the playdate is over. Their friends used to leave them with a big mess of toys and games to clean up. Now my children know to say, "Everyone needs to clean up." At first they felt weird about this, but when they remember that they won't want to have to clean up the entire mess alone (they know I'm not going to help, because I did not contribute to the mess), they speak up. When I know that the playdate is about to end, I give them a friendly reminder by asking, "Did you guys clean up?" This encourages my kids to get their friends involved in the cleanup before they walk out the door.

ANSWERS FROM ERICA'S EXPERT

Marianne Williamson is an internationally acclaimed spiritual teacher and bestselling author. Six of her ten published books have been *New York Times* best sellers. Four of these have been No. 1 *New York Times* best sellers. *A Return to Love* is considered a must-read of *The New Spirituality*. A paragraph from that book, beginning "Our deepest fear is not that we are inadequate. Our deepest fear is that we are powerful beyond measure..."—often misattributed to Nelson Mandela's inaugural address—is considered an anthem for a contemporary generation of seekers. Marianne's latest *New York Times* best seller is *A Course in Weight Loss: 21 Spiritual Lessons for Surrendering Your Weight Forever,* which was selected by Oprah to be one of her Favorite Things in 2010. Marianne's other books include *The Age of Miracles, Everyday Grace, A Woman's Worth, Illuminata, Healing the Soul of America,* and *The Gift of Change.* Marianne is a native of Houston, Texas. In 1989 she founded Project Angel Food, a meals-on-wheels program that serves homebound people with AIDS in the Los Angeles area. Today Project Angel Food serves more than a thousand people daily. In December 2006 a *Newsweek* magazine poll named her one of the fifty most influential baby boomers. Marianne has one daughter.

Disciplining with Love

What is the connection between spirituality and disciplining our children?

I think the goal is to model for our children the principles of the universe. On the one hand, the universe is infinite loving. On the other hand, there are consequences and the rule of Cause and Effect applies to everything we do. In the lives of children, as well as in the lives of adults, an infinitely loving universe is still best navigated with an intention and willingness to do the right thing.

What is a mother or father's role in disciplining their children?

Too many people today are afraid to parent; they end up underparenting, in my opinion. How would a small child know to say "hello," "please," and "thank you" unless someone taught them to—and yes, if necessary when they're very young, to insist that they do? Teaching our children manners is a gift to our children; it will serve them later on. No, as small children they don't understand why manners matter, but later in life they will be set up to win more, to succeed more, if they've developed that interpersonal skill. Same with getting enough sleep, telling the truth, not stealing or lying, cleaning up your room, working hard at school, playing well with others, and so forth. It's an unfair burden to place on children if we just leave those kinds of things up to the kids or expect them to possibly understand how deeply important such things will be for their entire lives. Discipline, when done with loving effectiveness, is a gift a parent gives a child.

How can you advise moms and dads to discipline their children from a spiritual perspective?

Discipline is not a bad word. We discipline best by modeling the discipline of love. But love does discipline. The ultimate goal is to cultivate in our children an organic gauge for right living, but until such a sense is fully developed within them, it's our job to guide their little ship.

And it always serves them to explain in age-appropriate language the why's of what we're asking them to do. "I'm insisting that you stay home this afternoon because you're tired and you're spinning out. I know you don't feel like you need a nap, but I'm your mom and I know that you do. And I know more about these things because I'm the adult and I'm your mom. I'm sorry if you're sad about this, and you're free to be sad about it. But you're staying home and resting, and I promise you you'll love your nap. And yes, I'll read you *The Bunny Book* again. Let's go find it now."

Is there anything wrong with saying no to your kids?

No! Love always gives the loving response, but sometimes the loving response in life is "No." Anyone who only says yes to their children is doing them a disservice, because one day that child will leave the parent's home and will encounter voices in the world that do say no. Teaching our children to respect appropriate authority is a gift to them, and when they're children, the authority is us (and the teacher at school and so forth). Lack of emotional and psychological training in navigating "no" as a child leads to brattiness, a sense of entitlement, a lack of ability to play on a team, and a lack of appropriate authority figures as an adult. That's usually not someone who's set up to succeed. Having said that, anytime we can say, "Yes, do this," rather than "No, don't do that," it's great. Someone told me that when my daughter was very young, and it was helpful advice. "Put the dishes in the sink, honey" is a much better directive than "Never leave dirty dishes on the counter."

Does our attitude as moms and dads impact how we discipline our children and how effective we are?

Of course. And that includes the understanding that we're in this situation to be the mother or the father, not to be the best friend.

How do you suggest teaching children about respect for others?

First and foremost, by explaining "why." It's best to start teaching the spiritual principles of life at a very young age. "You know, honey, everything we do comes back to us. Did you know that? If I'm nice to my friend, then my friend will be nicer to me! If I'm mean to my friend, my friend will be mean to me!"

PARENT: Did I see you take that ball from Joshua? Is that why he's crying?
CHILD: [Pouting]
PARENT: Honey, is that what happened? Why did you do that?
CHILD: I wanted it!
PARENT: Did Joshua know that?
CHILD: No.
PARENT: Then why didn't you tell him?
CHILD: I don't know.
PARENT: Well, if he didn't know and you just took it from him, then doesn't it
        make sense that he's crying? Wouldn't that make you cry, if someone
        did that to you?
CHILD: Yes . . .
PARENT: So let's go over and talk to Joshua, okay? Then you can tell him that
        you're sorry! Come on, honey. I'll go with you . . .

If you had the opportunity to raise your child all over again, is there anything that you would do differently?

First of all, I regret every moment I spent away from my daughter before she turned five. I totally understand now that before the age of five, everything we say and do goes directly into that little brain and becomes foundational. I didn't emotionally surrender to motherhood as much as I wish I had, and would do now if I had another chance.

What are some of the ways in which we can instill a sense of responsibility in our children?

By making it clear that they are responsible to us, and to the rest of their families. By making sure they behave responsibly toward other children, their clothes, their bodies, their rooms. The more we make these things operational from the time they're very small, the easier it all becomes later on. If you wait until the "eye-rolling years," it's hard to start in with the "You really shoulds . . ."

How can we apply spirituality in raising our children?

The best way to teach children spirituality is by making it situational.

- Pray with them before bedtime.
- Pray with them anytime they have a problem. "Oh, I know! Let's pray and ask God for a miracle!" And then do.
- Teach them forgiveness. "Well, if Jimmy was mean at school today, then he must be really sad. Maybe his house is sad or his Mommy and Daddy are sad. Let's pray for him!" And then do.
- Teach them to pray for healing. "Well, I'll take you to the doctor if you don't feel better soon. Right now, let's say a prayer and ask God to make your tummy stop hurting." And then do.

What are some parenting life lessons that you can pass along from your own experience?

I think the teen years are seriously risky in America today. No matter what socioeconomic neighborhood you live in, don't kid yourself: more often than you realize, there's crystal meth in the bathroom at the middle school. So I think there's a tendency for some of us to relax before it's safe to relax too much. Just because a child knows how to cross the street by him- or herself now, doesn't mean it's safe for them to do so. And girls should never go anywhere alone. They should always have at least one other girl with them. Even to the drugstore. In my case, at one point I trusted someone to take care of my daughter who I should not have trusted. When my daughter was little, I was obsessive about checking résumés, getting references, and so forth. But in the teen years I started to relax, and that was a mistake.

How can we discipline without feeling guilty?

You should only feel guilty if you're doing the wrong thing. Once you realize that proper, loving discipline is a loving thing to provide, then you don't feel guilty about it. And children would always have us feel guilty about making them do something they don't want to do. You have to learn to laugh at that, to tolerate their temporary hatred. It's one of those "you'll thank me later" moments.

Chapter 9

Nurture Your Child's Creativity

Make creative outlets and tools available to your children such as instruments, paints, paper, Lego, lessons, etc. Make opportunities and pay attention to their reactions. Encourage their creativity. Even do it with them. I always made sure there were musical instruments in the house. I made craft times available. I colored and danced around the house with [my son]. When he started showing interest in drums, I bought a cheap little plastic kit and when he was four, I put him in drum lessons.

—Pattie Mallette

When my kids were toddlers and preschoolers it was pretty easy to find creative things for them to do. Back then, drawing on a piece of paper and watching the color of the crayon or marker appear on the paper was exciting. Rolling, squeezing, and making shapes out of colored dough was something they enjoyed doing. (And, I admit, I did, too!) Back then I could also make up games for them to play and activities to do. For example, I took straws, cut them up, and then said, "Let's glue these on construction paper," and that was an exciting activity. And they loved board games. Favorites were Candy Land and Memory.

GO ON OUTINGS

I also tried to inspire creativity with simple outings. I'm not talking about outings far from home or that cost a lot of money. A simple walk around the block or to the corner can spark lots of interesting conversation and observations. Or go to a museum or local art gallery. Don't tell your kids where you're going; just tell them, "We're going out and when we get there I need you to help me find things." This makes it an exciting adventure and encourages them to notice the things around them. I did this often with Arianna and Addison, so that they could see and experience a variety of things and images and stimulate their minds. I'd pack lunch, so I was prepared for an unexpected stop in the park, and I tried to make it fun, engaging them by playing a game of I Spy at the museum or bringing markers and paper and having them sketch what they saw.

You don't have to spend hours at a museum—something that's not that appealing to young children. Even a quick visit offers benefits. Sometimes we'd go to the museum with the intention of just looking in the gift shop. And often those visits enticed us into a specific exhibit, because we'd see a T-shirt or book that interested us. I also tried to look for interactive exhibits— I remember one where the kids could sit in a bamboo raftlike object and float down a fake river—or those that contained things my kids loved, such as a helicopter on the ceiling.

In the car or on the walk back home, I'd ask my kids, "What did you like about that?" or "Do you want to go again?" Other times we'd get home and I'd tell them to draw what they'd seen.

BE CREATIVE WITH HOUSEHOLD ITEMS

Pots and pans are also great for younger children, such as preschoolers. These kitchen items can keep kids busy and safe while you are cooking or need to do something else around the house. Give them several pots and lids, and they can try to figure out which lid goes with which pot. They can also bang wooden spoons on the pots to make music. You can also fill up a plastic container with soapy water or let your kids make their own science project by adding ketchup, olive oil, beans, rice, etc., to a pot. Playing with pots and pans is a simple (and free) activity that's fun and allows your kids to be creative.

Even the most basic items around the house can spark a child's imagination. I remember one day, when my kids were a little younger, a box was delivered to our home with items I'd ordered. Once the box was empty, Addison got in it and Arianna pushed him around the house. Then they made a package out of it, and it became the "Where's Addison?" game. Just days later, Addison was drawing on this same box. It hung around the house for a week or two, and then I got rid of it.

MAKE CREATIVITY EASY

Now that my children are in grade school, it's sometimes not as easy to get them to do things that are creative. They're looking to be challenged and engaged. I've noticed that they don't pull out board games as much as they used to. I've tried rotating the games to different shelves, making some more visible than others, but this did not really help. I think that no matter how old your child is, it's more challenging to get them to do creative things when they're living in a world so consumed with technology. I don't have a problem with a little bit of technology, but it can be an overly independent activity. By this I mean that kids can be in their rooms playing video games and can become reclusive and cut off. To avoid this, when my kids are on their computers or using other forms of technology, I try to have them do so outside of their rooms. Instead, I have them use their devices in a room where we are all together, such as my office or the kitchen. I do this not just to monitor what they're viewing, but also so they are not isolated. Otherwise they risk becoming loners, feeling cut off, and instead of socializing with people they become more in tune with a device and not connected to another human spirit.

My kids need to be pushed a bit to be creative, so I try to make creativity easier and more accessible. We have this tiny art table in our kitchen with very small chairs from when the kids were little. I've squeezed it into the kitchen to encourage their creativity. I always keep paper, markers, and stickers on it. I've found that if I put these supplies up in a cabinet, my kids will never take them out, but if they're already visible, it encourages them to be expressive. Now they also draw and write on the table itself, and I don't mind because it's their art table. I also love to see what they come up with. Arianna enjoys writing, so she will make up a story, and Addison loves to draw, so he may make his own version of a book, things they didn't do when the stuff was put away.

I also keep creative projects nearby, such as a card-making kit, a stud kit, and fun supplies such as glue, fabric, and scissors. Often I have to be the one to push my kids to do creative things, but once they start, they really seem to enjoy it. It's important to teach our children how to sit still, enjoy the peace, and learn to entertain themselves.

BRING ON THE GAMES

My kids and I also play a lot of games together. Besides Uno, a card game that goes everywhere with us, I keep markers and paper in my purse, so when we go to a restaurant or are stuck in a waiting room they can draw or play Tic Tac Toe and Hangman. We'll also play I Spy, Would You Rather, and a game the kids made up called How Well Do You Know Me? (For this game, they pick one person in the room and have to say how well they know that person—for example, what's her favorite color, TV show, or food, or they have to answer questions such as would that person rather go to Italy or eat pizza or pasta.) We also cook and bake together to be creative.

Legos are a great tool for sparking creativity, not to mention helping kids with their fine motor skills. They're also something that kids play with for years and years and one of the few toys that seem to grow with them. Addison is obsessed with Legos, and I love seeing the creations he comes up with. Legos are also terrific because they come in various kits, from those that contain just pieces to those that give you instructions on how to build a specific object. Addison loves these, and I can see why. It's very challenging and satisfying to turn a bag full of Legos into something real you can play with, such as a car, firehouse, house, or character from a movie. Sometimes a kit is challenging and frustrating, but to me that's all part of the creative process.

ENCOURAGE THEIR PREFERENCES

When it comes to finding things my kids like to do now that they're a bit older, I've realized that it's important to pay attention to what your child loves to do creatively and to encourage that. Focus on what they're good at, *not* what you *want* them to be good at. There is a difference, and it's important to be aware of it. For example, you may want your child to play baseball, but if he'd rather build Legos, then help foster that. Or perhaps your daughter likes to paint her nails, as Arianna does. At first the smell drove me crazy, but I realized it was a creative outlet for her, so once I'd gotten her situated in a well-ventilated area and explained that she couldn't use nail polish in her bedroom, where she'd be inhaling it while she slept, I accepted that this was something creative she liked to do. (And something she's become quite good and innovative at, too. She recently came up with the idea of using toothpicks to put dots on her nails, and she now paints each one—fingers and toes—a different color.)

One way to help foster something your child loves to do is to research local classes. You will be surprised at what's out there. For example, because of Addison's patience and his strong attention to detail with Legos, I did a little research and found a robotics class for him in which they build Legos with batteries in them. I'd never heard of robotics until I did some digging, and it turns out to be a perfect match for him.

ENCOURAGE READING

Books are another way to get your kids into a creative mode, no matter how old they are. When my kids were toddlers, I never left the house without a book. There was always one in my diaper bag or stroller, and I'd pull it out and read it when we were on the go. Or we'd play a game with it where I'd ask my kids to find certain shapes, colors, or objects on the pages. I even brought waterproof books into the bathroom for bath time.

Something as simple as sitting on a park bench or in the tub with your child and a book can be surprisingly entertaining for both of you. For little ones, you don't always need a book to engage them. Just take a picture that's on your phone and ask them to point to certain things. As my kids have gotten older and learned to read, books have continued to be a great source of entertainment, as they can read to me or I can read to them.

ENCOURAGE WRITING

I also encourage Arianna to write in a journal. She sometimes has difficulties expressing her feelings or chooses not to express them verbally, so when she's upset I tell her to write down how she feels. I tell her that her journal is for her eyes only (and I stick to that), and that she should use it when she's mad or frustrated, as a release. I also tell her that she can write any words that come to mind—even curse words—so that she doesn't feel stifled. Everyone at every age needs a healthy release. It's about finding it and being able to go to it when you need it.

PLAY GAMES IN THE CAR

When we're in the car, I keep things entertaining and creative by introducing different games. My girlfriend's children taught us the game where you try to see how many out-of-state license plates you can spot. They also taught us a game in which you see how many different airlines you can name. You can also try to see how many street names you can think of or how many friends' addresses you can remember.

LET THEM DRESS THEMSELVES

I also believe in letting children wear what they want to wear. This may seem unrelated to the topic of creativity, but I feel it's part of learning freedom of expression. I don't try to control what my kids wear—even if it doesn't match. (I do, however, make sure it's appropriate for the weather and where we are going. For example, if we are going to a nice restaurant, they have to wear a decent outfit for that restaurant, not one they'd wear to the park.) Parents can have some control when we do our kids' shopping—I buy what I want my kids to have, what works for them, and what I think is appropriate—but when it's time to get dressed, it's their choice. Not only is it part of them being creative, but it also teaches them to make decisions. I encourage them to make their own decisions. It's their right.

They each have their own personal taste and style, and I support it. They know what they like and what they do not like. My daughter is at the age when I have to take her with me to try on clothing; I can't just assume something will fit her. She often grabs the things that she prefers, not necessarily what I prefer, and I let her do her thing. I interject only if an item is not appropriate.

CELEBRATE THEIR EFFORTS

When it comes to art your kids make, whether it's at school or home, I believe in hanging it up. You don't have to get an expensive frame or put it in a prominent spot in your home. But do tack it up somewhere. They'll feel proud about it, and it'll show them that you're not ashamed of it. I frame and hang all kinds of work. It keeps the memory of that time alive for each of us.

ANSWERS FROM ERICA'S EXPERT

Here, my fifth-grade teacher, Jan Schlossberg, answers more questions, this time on nurturing a child's creativity. As a teacher for thirty years, she has a lot of wisdom to impart.

Creative Kids

With the rapid advances in technology and so much available to our children today, what effects do you see on children (positive and negative)?

This is an exciting time to grow up. Our children are more sophisticated and informed, because technology allows them to find answers instantly. Children are more technologically savvy. This is clearly a good thing. Computer programs often encourage analytical thinking. Many programs encourage creative and open-ended thinking. As a teacher, I often use the computer to enhance my teaching.

What impact do you think technology can have on our children's creativity?

I think that it is extremely important for a child to experience painting firsthand with paint, brush, and paper. Primary experiences with artistic material are extremely important for a young child's development. Playing with clay, colorfully textured paper, and bright colored pens allow the child to mess around. This type of open-ended thinking has no "right or wrong" answer. If the child wants to create a purple triangular pumpkin, he can. I also believe, however, that technology does encourage creative thought. For example, there are amazing architectural programs that encourage design, form, shape, and function. There are many lovely writing programs that set the framework for great writing.

As with everything in life, computers must be used with discretion. Using them as the only source for creative thinking, however, is a questionable choice. For balance, a child needs both the primary experience and the technological challenge.

How can parents regulate their kids' technology so that they don't isolate themselves?

Parents must be keenly aware when their young child is on the computer. For the first ten years of my children's lives, they were allowed to use *only* the family room computer. I was always watching, and they knew where they could travel on the Internet. We had many conversations about the dangers of the Internet. As my sons grew, so did their latitude and responsibility. I allowed computers in their rooms, but with the following rule: all doors must be open. They were keenly aware of the consequences if they betrayed my trust.

There has to be a commonsense approach. Growing children should play team sports, tennis, or golf. They should have playdates. They should run and skip and play in the sand. They should go to movies and read lots of books. They should not be on the computer for an unspecified amount of time. I would never allow a young child to own a BlackBerry. Unsupervised use of the Internet is fraught with problems. Communication is the key. Initiate important guidelines. Make sure there is no gray area. Be clear and concise. If your child violates the agreed-upon rules, there should be consequence of merit. In other words, take away a special toy or dessert. Then, once again, talk. The conversation after the punishment is crucial. Then hug and kiss your child. He will leave the experience understanding what it means to lose a parent's trust. He will also understand that he is loved deeply.

What are some of the best ways to nurture your child's creativity if the child is a toddler or preschooler?

With very young children, everything should be hands-on and experiential. For example, if you are introducing the color yellow, you can bring in a large bowl of lemons and bananas. The child should be able to play with the yellow fruit and then taste it. Finger paint with the color yellow, play with yellow Play-Doh, cook yellow pudding or corn bread, and drink lemonade—all these activities not only support the concept of yellow, but also allow for spontaneity and creativity. Providing the child with free exploration with a variety of tactile activities allows for creativity.

Additionally, I am a *huge* proponent of classical music. I support playing Mozart, Bach, or Vivaldi as background to create a curious mind. The complexity of the musical notes spurs on brain activity. It also warms the heart.

What are some of the best ways to nurture your child's creativity if the child is in the younger grades in elementary school, such as kindergarten and first grade?

What is creativity? It is open-ended thinking with no right answer. Creative thought has been called divergent thinking. Creativity involves thinking. For young children, an atmosphere of openness must be created. In the primary grades, children need to learn many aspects of creativity. Teaching the child how to distinguish between the figure and the background is an important developmental skill. Often the child will scribble a picture with one color. Slowly, with lots of activities, the child will begin to distinguish the dog from the park background. While you work on this skill, you can simultaneously allow for creativity. During Halloween, I often ask my students to create a square purple pumpkin with jewels for eyes. Why do pumpkins always have to be orange and round? I will ask them to create a magic pencil that can do magical things. Young children also need the free flow of experiences. Finger painting is a great medium. Pudding is fun to finger paint with; green shaving cream before St. Patrick's Day creates lots of giggles. Inventiveness nurtures creative thinking. Ribbons, stickers, straws, plastic trays, cardboard tubes, and other items that would normally be tossed away can be recycled into the best inventions.

What are some of the best ways to nurture your child's creativity if she is in an older grade, such as third, fourth, or fifth?

Creativity doesn't occur in a vacuum. It is a type of thinking that has structure. Teaching the older child this structure gives her a "road map" to the creative process. Asking the child to "create" is unfair in some ways. You begin with the brainstorming process. Let's take the same problem of changing an ordinary pencil into something else. You actively brainstorm all your ideas on a dry-erase board. Just get the child's ideas out there. There should be no evaluation at this point. After you have filled the board with ideas, take another colorful pen and circle the ideas you love the most. Erase everything else. Fine-tune this list until you have your top two or three ideas. If you are asking the child to write about his new invented pencil, then write the topic at the top of the page. Then start listing the details of this idea. Next, encourage elaboration of this same idea. Lots of description will bring the ideas to life.

Brainstorming, evaluation, and elaboration comprise the process that encourages creativity. In his Structure of Intellect model, Dr. J. P. Guilford delineated this model for creative thought. It is unfair to ask the older child to "write." Repeatedly using this creative process helps give structure to creative thought.

Chapter 10

Nurture Your Child's Giving Heart

My mottoes are "Service is the rent you pay for living" and "To whom much is given, much is expected." And I use every opportunity to teach these important lessons to my children because I believe that they are never too young to hear about volunteerism, and that you must raise grateful and giving children. My kids know that when they receive a gift, they must donate a gift. They've traveled to the most impoverished countries in the world, so when they complain and I say to be grateful for your blessings, it immediately hits home.

—Malaak Compton-Rock, mother of three

A few years ago when my daughter was about eight years old, the two of us were wrapping Christmas gifts. I had bought one of my sisters a wallet. I didn't know if she needed a wallet, but I knew she was planning to travel out of the country.

"I know what," I said out loud, talking to myself. "I'm going to put some euros in this wallet." I didn't even think Arianna had heard me—until a few minutes later.

"Mommy, I want to put some money in it, too, because I know things are bad right now," she said, referring to the grim economy she had heard me talking about. "I want to give Auntie some of my own money."

"Okay," I said. I was touched. It was sweet. Then she went to her room and returned a few minutes later hiding her hands behind her back. I'd figured she'd gotten a dollar or two.

"Mom, don't say a word. I want to do this on my own without you telling me what I can give or knowing how much," she said. "I'm giving what my heart is telling me to give."

"You don't have to hide it," I told her. "This is your thing and I promise I'm not going to say anything." So she handed me the money: forty-five dollars she'd taken from her piggy bank. I was amazed and proud, because one message I'd always tried to give my children was that they have to share what they have. I want to raise them with a spirit of giving, a spirit that I hope will be part of them their entire lives. I try not to tell them what to give or to judge them for what they give. Giving is giving.

I also try to explain that whatever they receive, whether it's a dollar or clothing, they need to share with those who are less fortunate. For example, when I buy my kids a brand-new pair of shoes, they know to come home and find a pair to give away. I let them pick which shoes to donate, and I don't say no, whether it's a pair that has been worn or a pair that's brand-new. I want it to be their choice. The same goes for money, whether it is cash they get as part of their allowance each Saturday, on a holiday, or for a birthday, or money they've earned. I call it the three S's: share, save, and spend. And this is the order in which I encourage them to remember when it comes to money. I want to teach them to think of someone else first.

When they were younger, we had a plastic jar in the kitchen that we called our family's "Share Jar." Each one of us contributed money to the jar and then we gave that money to a charity of our choice or to someone in need, such as a homeless man on the street. Now that they're older, the Share Jar has turned into a Share Envelope, but the concept is the same. I never tell them how much to share or whom to give the money to. I just want them to appreciate all that they have been given and to share with others.

Sometimes, after my daughter has received money, she will hand some to me and say, "Mommy, I want to send this money to Africa," or after a big disaster, such as the 2010 earthquake in Haiti or the recent one in Japan, both kids have come to me with money to donate or have contributed it to a fund-raiser at their school. When Arianna was younger, she thought this "sharing" included her brother. I remember one time her going up to him and saying, "Here's a dollar for you. I want to share this money." Other times, they'll want to share it with their grandmother (my mother), or they'll just give me some money without saying whom they want to give it to. Another time, when Addison was five or six years old, he handed me two dollars and said the money was for his friends who are twin boys. I saved that money in an envelope until I saw the mom, which was about six months later.

I started donating when my kids were babies, but I brought this awareness to them about sharing when they were about two or three years old. At that age, they may be too little to understand, but I don't think it's ever too young to start talking to our kids about the world outside of them.

Another thing we do regularly is send packages of our things to a village in Africa. I found out about it when my daughter was in kindergarten and we did a charity walk through her school. The charity was raising money for an organization in Kenya, and the man in charge of it walked with us. I told him that I wanted to help his village, so we exchanged information and I've been sending boxes there ever since. A few times a year I'll fill a box (any size) with our gently used items such as clothes, shoes, books, markers, pens, coloring books, backpacks, games, and pajamas. (We do not send clothes that are torn or damaged or toys and games that are useless.) Like many kids in this country, my kids have way too much (more than I had at their age), and I want them to start early to think of others.

When my kids were much younger, I gathered some of what we were going to donate while they were taking naps or at school. I did a big sweep of their toys and games, weeding out the items I knew they didn't remember they had or that they hadn't touched in eons. Doing some of this donating while they were sleeping or at school prevented them from getting too attached to items they didn't truly want, but just didn't want to part with.

This was just the beginning for me because I'd also involve them in the rest of the donating, saying, "We're going to clean out. Go in your rooms and find things to donate." This continues to be part of our donating ritual. They gather up whatever they want to contribute. Sometimes they get attached to items—even clothes that don't fit. Addison got upset when I wanted to donate a favorite pair of his sneakers that didn't fit him anymore. We had gotten him new shoes, so I told him he had to pass along the old ones. "Donate any other shoes," he told me, "but not those." I was fine with that. At times like that I remind my kids that another boy or girl who has far less than they do really needs these items. I have to say things such as "We're going to give this stuff to people who don't have as much and who really need it. It might put a smile on their faces and warm their hearts." This usually works. Other times, I'm amazed at their generosity as they donate a toy or item they recently got and adored, or hand me a whole bunch of items to add to the box. They may not have understood much about what we were doing when they were toddlers, but by the time they were four or five years old, donating became such a normal part of their lives.

Sometimes during the year my kids will randomly hand me something, even when I'm not putting a box together, and say, "I want to donate this." I send the boxes directly to that man I met at the charity walk, and he shares them with the village. I like sending donations there because I know exactly where they're going. What's helped my kids want to share their things is that the man we send them to writes us letters and includes pictures of the kids in Africa wearing the items we passed on to them. This makes it very concrete for them. Rather than their having to imagine that their clothes and toys are going to this great unknown place, they actually see a photo of a child wearing Addison's pajamas or Arianna's shoes. They also see how frail the kids are and how the children their age are swimming in their clothes because the clothes are so big on them. Or they see a boy wearing Arianna's shoes or an eleven-year-old wearing the clothes that fit Addison when he was just five. Sometimes we'll even get photos of adults wearing my kids' clothes, and that shows us with how little these people have, how they have to make whatever they get work. It helps remind them about all that they do have and the blessings they've been given. It also makes them feel good to help others and to know that perhaps if they hadn't given that boy shoes, he may not have anything to wear at all. I remind Arianna and Addison of this often. I want them to think of themselves and take great care of themselves and all the things that they have, but also to know it is as important to share with those in need. Through this process, my kids are not only learning about donating. They are also learning about and seeing the process of recycling.

ANSWERS FROM ERICA'S EXPERT

Once again, my wonderful former fifth-grade teacher, Jan Schlossberg, has some terrific insight into this topic of nurturing your child's giving heart and teaching him about volunteering.

Getting Kids to Care

What are some ways to get grade-schoolers involved with volunteering?

Teaching compassion begins at an early age. Use Thanksgiving, Christmas, and Hanukkah as a springboard to giving back. You can systematically clean the child's room with him. "How about giving all your old books and toys to children who don't have many toys?" Take your child with you as you turn in his toys. Let him see where his toys are going. In Los Angeles, there is an organization called MEND, Meet Each Need with Dignity. Food and new clothing are given to the needier families in our neighborhoods. Every city has organizations like this.

One of my students created an organization called Books and Blankies. She made small quilts and created a book drive at our school. She and her mom delivered these books and blankets to schools. This drive was hugely successful, and my student learned a life lesson. Other children are not as fortunate as she is.

Giving back can take many forms. Besides tangible items, it can mean volunteering time to animal rescue organizations, senior citizen homes, hospitals, food banks, and rescue missions—organizations that need human beings helping other human beings. It is my belief that a child as young as five can begin to understand what giving back means. Taking a child to an animal rescue place helps create empathy. Bringing along blankets and food helps the child begin to realize that animals are helpless victims that need our help.

What are some ways to get grade-schoolers involved in volunteering?

Most elementary schools are involved with charity organizations and volunteering. World catastrophes such as the earthquake in Haiti and the tsunami in Japan are important events to respond to. A Daisy troop selling Girl Scout cookies to raise money for the Red Cross is a great way to get the child involved in helping others. Often schools have sister schools that need help with creating better libraries, putting computers in the classroom, getting books for an entire class, and other noteworthy endeavors.

Habitat for Humanity is an amazing organization that would appeal to sixth- and seventh-graders. Raising money for a Seeing Eye dog, however, can happen in kindergarten. Sadly, there is so much suffering in our world that it is easy to find an organization that needs help.

Is there an age that's too young to get children involved in volunteering or charity?

I think that five years old is the perfect age to begin developing an understanding of charity and giving back. Younger children are appropriately self-involved and see the world through their young needs and wants. At age five, the child is just beginning to see beyond his own needs.

For disasters such as those in Haiti and Japan, was there anything you noticed at your school or did with your students to contribute to these causes?

Absolutely. My school immediately began fund-raising for the victims in Haiti and Japan. Besides fund-raising, our students wrote letters to children in these two countries. There is an organization called Generosity Water, which builds water wells in developing countries. We raised enough money to build two wells. The children were bringing in their piggy banks, doing extra chores, and selling lemonade to help earn money for this organization.

Do you think pen pals are helpful tools for kids to learn about the world outside of them. What is the benefit?

Over the years, my students have had pen pals, and I thought the experiences were noteworthy. Often relationships were formed that were touching. There are other ways to create these types of relationships, however. One example is by using the book by Jeff Brown, *Flat Stanley*. This is a charming story about a little boy, named Stanley Lambchop, who was flattened by a falling bookcase. At first his family was extremely upset, but eventually they began to realize that being flat had its virtues. He could travel easily and have lots of cool adventures. Using *Flat Stanley* as our vehicle, we wrote to other schools around America who were also having fun with Stanley. There is even a *Flat Stanley* website, flatterworld.com, which allows other schools to contact your school. This year, we wrote to schools in Kaplan, Louisiana; Austin, Texas; and New York. We wrote letters, drew pictures about Southern California, took photos of our school, and let them have a glimpse into our lives. They did the same thing for us. We learned about Mardi Gras, crayfish, and the Gulf of Mexico. We would chart all the places we communicated with on a big U.S. map. Mostly the students learned that the other students were very much like them. It was really a sensational adventure. The children learned about our country's geography, and about how other people live. This is an adventure that we will definitely repeat.

Using the *Flat Stanley* experience is an amazing way to introduce the world to your child. You can do this on your own. Your child can create his own Stanley and send it to children in other parts of the world. Get a large map of the world. This is an experience that is so wonderful.

Giving heart is a wonderful term. How do I make use of it?

Giving heart is so important. I begin by letting the children observe who I am as a person and as a teacher. I share my heart daily with my young charges. I often begin each day with visualization. I ask the children to visualize a beautiful satin box with a lovely ribbon. Then I ask them to visualize peeking inside. At this point, I ask them to open their eyes. I have a satin box open with sparkling glitter inside. Inside is "today." I sprinkle the glitter around the children, sharing with them that today is the "gift" you give yourself. It is yours to do as you wish. If you wish to have a magical day, you will. If you wish to have a grumpy day, then chances are you will. Having a grumpy day is okay, but it is important to teach that it is a choice.

Giving heart means expressing your truest feelings and teaching the children to do the same. Teaching by example is called "modeling." Modeling how to communicate in a kind manner, expressing kindness just to be kind, doing acts of kindness—all are important lessons for youngsters to observe. We need to stimulate their minds and their hearts. That is what good parents and teachers do.

Chapter 11

LoveKids

The role of a mother never ends and always changes. My daughter, Kirby, is twenty-two, and my son, Will, is twenty-one. When they were young, I focused on the basics: right and wrong, manners, kindness, and being responsible. I know children absorb every move you make, so I was aware of my own actions and the messages they send. As they got older, they no longer needed me the same way. It's a big transition, but to this day I continue to bombard them with love and advice (sometimes unsolicited). They still value my opinion, and the good news is I'm still just as interested in hearing theirs. The true definition of success for me is children who grow up to be healthy, happy, compassionate, and thinking human beings. There is nothing more important.

—Gayle King, mother of two

The other morning, when I realized that my children had missed the school bus, I started to cry. I literally slid down the wall to the floor (like you see in the movies) and sat there with big, fat tears streaming down my face. It sounds a little silly to me now, days later and with a clearer head, but it was a huge shining lightbulb moment for me. I realized, no matter what I do for others every day, I still exist and I need to find and connect with the person, the woman, again. Otherwise, my full plate will only spell out "stress," and I will ignore my own health and only preach about it for others. None of us is perfect and all our journeys are a work in progress—mine, too. Just because I have written this book about my journey doesn't mean it's over.

The reason for my stress that day was a combination of things: I hadn't worked out in months because of a minor taxi accident, so I had had no stress release; my husband's career was in transition; and I was busy with school committees. On top of all that, I was a full-time mom without full-time child care, so I was busy tending to my children's daily emotional and physical needs, *and* I was nearing the deadline for this book. I had been working on it for hours each day, and when I was not working on it, I was thinking about it. Why? Because my hope is that I am creating something that can help others. The whole point of this book is to make a contribution to the lives of the innocent: our children. My hope is that someone's life can be impacted by even just one of the simple things I share in these pages, because often one simple thing can end up being a big thing in your life and the life of your children.

Looking back on my journey, which started the day Addison was lying sick on the bathroom floor, I realize what a long journey it has been and how far my children have come. I am so thankful for the experience, because when I really think about all I went through, I know it happened for a reason, and that was to share what I learned with you. Don't get me wrong, it still hurts, really hurts, to think about Addison in the hospital. But it is not a hurt that handicapped me. It is a hurt that made me do something. It made me learn from the experience, the moment and the trauma of it all. It gave me an awareness that I am using to benefit him, my family, and hopefully you.

I'm so grateful to have both of my children alive and healthy. I'm also beyond happy that I allowed my inner voice to be my guide when I started this journey. At the time of Addison's illness, I was just a young mom going up against experts, people who had years of hands-on experience and training, with what I had brought to them. What really made this journey a success was intuition—embracing it, loving it, and using it. After that, everything else fell into place. As much as you want to give up and second-guess that inner voice, don't do it. That voice is there for a reason. It is there to guide you, especially as you navigate life as a mother, father, or caregiver of a child.

When I got married and became a mother, I was clueless. It was *all* new to me, and I was at home alone trying to figure it out while my husband was at work. I believe I had the confidence to embark on this journey because, prior to all this, I spent many hours watching *Oprah* during the late '90s. (That was my free therapy.) It was during this time that I began to embrace my being and work on myself, because I knew something big was coming my way. I knew one day I was going to be a mom. But in order for me to be the mom and the person I desired, I had to work on myself. I had to heal myself, and I needed to be fulfilled, but I had no guidance on how to get there, other than Oprah. But I also had my inner voice. That voice was my guide. We all possess it. Let's use it!

Birthing a child or being fortunate enough to have one come from the heart is a blessing. We asked for this child, so now what? We have a serious responsibility when bringing the innocent into the world. It is our duty to provide them with more beyond the basics of food, shelter, and clothing. Our children are not ours; they are ours to borrow. We are the vessel used to bring them to life.

Our job, our responsibility, is to expose our children and learn with them, but also *for* them! Bringing awareness is a constant, ever-moving journey, one that we decided to embark on the day we shifted roles from men and women to fathers and mothers, or caregivers. Learn your options, and work to make life better for you and your children. Explore and have lots of faith and *believe*. Enjoy these years.

With much love and support,

Erica

Really Easy Recipes Your Kids Will Love

We as adults need to come together and provide useful and realistic information for our children today. We have to teach them about portion control, how to avoid processed foods, and how to create balanced meals made of clean, beautiful foods. It's also crucial to have mealtime together whenever possible. We are the example and we set the tone. Let's make a real effort to make the kitchen table a healthy place to come together.

—Ricki Lake, mother of two

From what you've read so far in this book, it may sound like I am some sort of cook. I'm not. Before Addison was hospitalized, I used to hate cooking. I felt as if I cooked all day only to make food that was eaten in minutes. I hated being in the kitchen—which is why having a chapter full of recipes is even a surprise to me. But once I started this journey, I knew that preparing our own food was part of improving my family's health. At first I didn't like it. I hated washing and chopping. Most of my friends said cooking was fun because they'd sip wine while they did it, and they actually made it look cool with their snacks and pretty glasses of wine. But I don't drink and I didn't have one of those big chef's kitchens you see on TV. What motivated me to get in the kitchen and stay there was the fact that I wanted my kids to eat healthy. It felt good to feed them the fresh meals I'd cooked. I also discovered the excitement, curiosity, and challenge of seeing all these different ingredients and figuring out what I could do with them. Today, I see cooking somewhat like a science experiment, and I get through by thinking about the end result.

Through this process, I've realized two things: First, I don't have to make recipes that take hours, consist of complicated steps, or require a lot of fancy appliances and kitchen tools. I can go in the kitchen, make easy, healthy meals, and call it a day. Second, it is satisfying to create meals my family loves, foods that are truly benefiting their health. It actually makes it more enjoyable and worth it. And so does the thumbs-up I get from husband and kids when I make a new recipe. (The occasional two thumbs-up is really satisfying!)

I've also made cooking work for me, my family, and my busy schedule by preparing a lot of things in bulk one day a week. This takes a few hours on that one day, but then lunch and dinner take just minutes to pull together. You don't have to be a gourmet chef or a cook of any sort. Just go in the kitchen and experiment. Also, your children don't have to be sick for you to think of food in a healing, healthful way. By giving them fresh, nutritious foods, you're starting good habits and giving them the vitamins and nutrients they need to grow.

What follows are simple recipes for the clean, lean food I make for my family. None of these recipes take very long or require much skill. And none contain dairy, white flour, eggs, sugar, table salt, or nuts. They're recipes I came up with that my family loves and that have kept us all satisfied and healthy. What more could you ask for?

COOKING TIPS

A few general tips that go with many of the recipes that follow:

- When adding seasoning to a dish, season the pan first. By this I mean put the pan on the stove, turn on the heat, and, while it's warming up, add the seasoning directly to the pan before adding the main ingredients such as tofu or fish.
- Many of the recipes here call for seasonings such as umeboshi vinegar, Sea Veg (Maine Coast Sea Vegetables is the brand I use), lemon juice, and lime juice. The amount listed in each recipe is a recommended amount. I suggest seasoning to taste.
- Ingredients such as Sea Veg, umeboshi vinegar, and kombu are available at most health food stores, in the Japanese aisle. Other ingredients, such as agave and manuka honey, can be found at the health food store.
- For recipes requiring a pan, use a cast-iron pan, but any frying pan or skillet will do.

Mother's Love Recipes

ENTREES

Sunday Chicken

I made this chicken one Sunday, and the result was two thumbs-up from my kids. Now it's part of our family's repertoire of favorite dishes. Serve it with brown or jasmine rice along with a veggie for a nice, well-rounded meal. After cooking the chicken, save the juice that's in the pan. It's delicious over rice and great to drizzle on leftover chicken the next day when you're heating it up. It will add moisture and flavor.

Serves 4

Ingredients
1 whole chicken (organic if possible), rinsed
6 sprigs fresh rosemary
6 garlic cloves, sliced in half
¼ cup extra-virgin olive oil
⅔ cup fresh-squeezed lime juice (about 4 limes)
3 tablespoons fresh-squeezed lemon juice (about 1 lemon)
⅛ teaspoon sea salt
¼ teaspoon Sea Veg
½ teaspoon mirin (rice cooking wine)
5 sprigs fresh thyme
1 teaspoon oregano

1. Preheat oven to 350°F.
2. Scrape any excess yellow fat off the chicken skin with a knife. Place the chicken, breast side up, into a medium-size glass casserole dish.
3. Place 1 rosemary sprig in the dish and sprinkle half the garlic cloves on the chicken.
4. Whisk together the olive oil, lime juice, lemon juice, sea salt, Sea Veg, the leaves of 3 rosemary sprigs, and the mirin. Drizzle mixture over the chicken.

5. Place remaining 2 rosemary sprigs, the thyme, and oregano around the chicken in the baking dish.

6. Cover the chicken loosely with foil to keep it moist. The foil shouldn't cover the corners of the baking dish.

7. Cook for 1 hour and 30 minutes, basting the chicken 3 times so it doesn't dry out.

8. Remove the foil and cook for an additional 45 minutes, basting chicken about 5 times. (I increase the amount of basting here to keep it moist and prevent any burning.)

9. For the last 5 minutes, turn the oven to broil or 500°F. This gives the chicken a beautiful golden, crispy appearance. (It's so pretty you won't want to cut it!)

Random Chicken

This recipe came about when I needed to make dinner and randomly grabbed different ingredients from the cabinets and my refrigerator, trying to figure out what to make. I experimented as I went along.

Serves 4

Ingredients

1 whole chicken (organic, if possible), rinsed

⅓ cup extra-virgin olive oil

½ teaspoon Sea Veg

2 bay leaves

½ teaspoon garlic powder

½ teaspoon poultry seasoning

1 teaspoon Italian seasoning

⅓ cup fresh-squeezed lime juice (about 2 limes)

2 tablespoons fresh-squeezed lemon juice (about 1 lemon)

1. Preheat oven to 350°F.
2. Scrape any excess yellow fat off the chicken skin with a knife.
3. Drizzle 3 tablespoons of the oil into a glass baking dish. Place chicken breast side up; sprinkle ¼ teaspoon Sea Veg and the bay leaves inside the chicken.
4. Turn the chicken over and sprinkle ¼ teaspoon garlic powder, ¼ teaspoon poultry seasoning, and ½ teaspoon Italian seasoning on the other side.
5. Return chicken to breast side up. Pour the remaining oil over the top. Add the lime and lemon juices, the remaining Sea Veg, garlic powder, poultry seasoning, and Italian seasoning.
6. Place a loose-fitting piece of foil over bird and bake 1 ½ to 2 hours.
7. Baste chicken 3 times to keep it moist. (Smaller birds may need an addition of 1 cup water in the baking dish due to low fat content.)
8. Remove foil after 1 ½ to 2 hours, and bake 30 additional minutes. For the last 5 minutes, turn the oven to 500°F or to broil. This crisps up the skin, giving it a golden appearance.

Trying Tofu

This recipe is an easy way to get kids to eat tofu. Mine love it. Just make sure to get your pan hot first; then add the oil and tofu pieces. This prevents the tofu from sticking.

Serves 4

Ingredients

14-ounce package extra-firm tofu, rinsed

2 ½ tablespoons soy sauce (gluten-free or wheat-free variety, but you can use regular soy sauce, too)

3 tablespoons extra-virgin olive oil

¼ teaspoon Sea Veg

1. Cut the tofu into 9 equal pieces. Place on a double-layered paper towel to drain for 10 minutes.
2. Heat a large skillet on low heat. Add 2 tablespoons oil, 1 ½ tablespoons soy sauce, and ⅛ teaspoon Sea Veg.
3. Place well-drained tofu slabs into the pan, allowing enough room between the pieces so you can turn them over easily.
4. Drizzle remaining oil, soy sauce, and Sea Veg on top of tofu. Turn heat up to medium and pan-fry 3 to 5 minutes on each side, until golden.

Soy Sauce Salmon

I buy wild salmon and try to get the thin fillets. Just make sure to rinse the salmon well before cooking. I usually leave the skin on while cooking, but you can take it off, if you prefer.

Serves 4

Ingredients

    2 tablespoons extra-virgin olive oil

    2 tablespoons soy sauce (gluten-free, wheat-free, but you can use regular soy sauce, too)

    ¼ teaspoon Sea Veg

    4 thin wild salmon fillets or 1 pound wild salmon cut into 4 pieces

1. Heat a medium-size skillet on low. Add 1 tablespoon oil, 1 tablespoon soy sauce, and sprinkle ⅛ teaspoon Sea Veg.
2. Add the salmon pieces, skin side down. Cook 3 to 5 minutes.
3. Drizzle the remaining oil, soy sauce, and Sea Veg on top of fish.
4. Turn salmon over, cover, and cook 3 to 5 minutes. (Depending on how thick the salmon is and how well-done you prefer it, cook it longer if you like it well-done, shorter if you like it rarer.)

Grey Sole

My kids really enjoy grey sole with a side of beans or a vegetable such as kale. Sometimes I'll take a piece of nori, spread on white or short-grain brown rice (not sushi rice), and add the grey sole. Then I roll it like a burrito and cut it into pieces for my own version of sushi.

Serves 2

Ingredients

½ pound grey sole, left whole or cut into 2 pieces
2 tablespoons extra-virgin olive oil, plus some to drizzle over fillets
½ lemon cut into three wedges
2 fresh thyme sprigs
4 pinches Sea Veg
3 pinches ground, dried thyme

1. Rinse the fish and place on a paper towel to dry.
2. Add the oil to a medium-size skillet and squeeze in the juice of 2 lemon wedges. Gently heat over a low flame. Place 1 thyme sprig on each side of the pan.
3. Add 2 pinches Sea Veg to middle of pan. Place fish fillets, serving side down, between the two thyme sprigs and season top of the fish with a drizzle of oil; the juice of 1 lemon wedge; ground, dried thyme; and remaining Sea Veg.
4. Cook for 2 to 3 minutes. Gently turn fillets over and cook 2 minutes.

Baked Cod

This is another fish recipe that my family really enjoys. It's so simple it takes barely any time to make.

Serves 4

Ingredients
1 ¼ pounds cod, cut into 4 equal pieces
1 tablespoon plus 1 teaspoon extra-virgin olive oil
½ teaspoon Sea Veg
2 tablespoons fresh lemon juice (about 1 lemon)
4 thin slices lemon
1 ½ cups shredded carrots

1. Preheat oven to 350°F.
2. Rinse cod and place on a paper towel to dry.
3. Drizzle 1 tablespoon oil, ⅛ teaspoon Sea Veg, and 1 tablespoon lemon juice into a glass baking dish. Add the cod, serving side up.
4. Season fish with 1 teaspoon oil and remaining Sea Veg and lemon juice. Place one slice of lemon on each piece of cod. Add the carrots around the fish pieces.
5. Cover the dish with foil and place in the oven. Bake for 15 to 20 minutes.

Chicken Strips

These are great for a birthday party or any other gathering. They're pretty simple to make. I use a brown paper bag to shake the flour mixture and the raw chicken together, because it coats it quickly and evenly, but the bag is optional. You can also put the brown rice flour and Sea Veg mix in a bowl and roll the chicken pieces in it.

Serves 4

Ingredients

1 ½ cups brown rice flour
2 ½ teaspoons Sea Veg
1 cup extra-virgin olive oil
½ cup fresh lemon juice (about 3 lemons)
1 pound boneless, skinless chicken breasts, rinsed, pounded ¼-inch thick, sliced into 4-inch-by-2-inch strips

1. Mix flour and Sea Veg in a doubled-up brown paper bag.
2. Combine ¼ cup oil and the lemon juice. Dip chicken pieces in this, coating on both sides; then drop into paper bag. Shake well. Lift chicken out, gently shaking off excess flour. Set aside on a plate.
3. Heat a large skillet with half the remaining oil on medium heat. Add half the chicken pieces and cook 3 to 4 minutes, until lightly golden. Turn the pieces over and cook another 3 minutes. Drain on paper towels.
4. Add remaining oil and fry second batch of chicken. Drain well.

VEGETABLE SIDES

Steamed Broccoli

Whenever I serve this to my children's friends, I usually get a call from their mothers the next day. They say that their children came home telling them they had to make "Addison's mom's broccoli" or "Arianna's mom's broccoli." These moms can't believe their children ate broccoli, and so much of it! Once I give them the recipe, they're shocked at how easy it is to make. You can also make this with steamed cauliflower or carrots, or all three veggies in a bowl together.

Serves 4

Ingredients

1 bunch broccoli, cleaned in cold water with a tablespoon of sea salt, rinsed well

2 teaspoons flaxseed oil

Juice of ½ lemon

1. Remove broccoli stems, leaving three inches under the florets. Cut into bite-size pieces. Place in a steamer basket. Set into a large pot with 2 cups water. Bring to boil and steam 3 to 5 minutes, until broccoli is bright green.
2. Remove broccoli and place in a bowl. Drizzle flaxseed oil and lemon juice. Stir and serve.

Baked Lemon-Garlic Broccoli

This delicious side dish goes perfectly with tofu, fish, or chicken. It's also good on top of brown rice pasta.

Serves 4

Ingredients

　　1 bunch broccoli, cleaned in cold water with a tablespoon of sea salt, rinsed well

　　2 tablespoons extra-virgin olive oil

　　½ cup fresh-squeezed lemon juice (about 3 lemons)

　　3 garlic cloves, cut finely

　　Pinch sea salt

　　1 tablespoon flaxseed oil (optional)

1. Preheat oven to 350°F.
2. Remove broccoli stems, leaving three inches under the florets. Cut into bite-size pieces. Put in medium-size baking dish. Drizzle with oil and lemon juice. Sprinkle with garlic.
3. Bake 10 minutes, pull out of the oven, and flip pieces once. Bake additional 10 minutes until edges are lightly browned.
4. When done, sprinkle lightly with sea salt. Drizzle with flaxseed oil, if using. (Don't bake flaxseed oil or you will damage its nutrients.)

Steamed Green Peas

Like the broccoli, this gets raves from my kids and their friends. It also makes a great baby food—just skip the flaxseed oil and puree peas in a blender.

Serves 4

Ingredients

10-ounce package frozen green peas (preferably organic)
1 ½ teaspoons flaxseed oil

1. Place peas in a steamer basket. Add to a small pot with 1 cup water. Bring to a boil.
2. Steam for 3 to 5 minutes, or until peas are bright green and tender in the middle.
3. Remove peas from the steamer basket and place in a serving bowl. Stir in the flaxseed oil and serve.

Steamed Leafy Greens

I make this with a variety of leafy greens, such as kale and collard greens. Whichever leafy greens you choose, make sure to soak them in a bowl of cold water with a tablespoon of sea salt for several minutes, changing the water until it's clean and gently scrubbing the leaves with your hand. The salt helps remove any tiny bugs from the leaves.

Serves 6

Ingredients

1 bunch leafy greens (kale or collard greens) torn into bite-size pieces, stems removed
Umeboshi vinegar (to taste)

1. Place leafy greens in a steamer basket in a large pot with 2 cups water. Bring to a boil.
2. Steam for 3 to 5 minutes or until bright green and tender.
3. Remove greens from steamer and place in a serving bowl. Add the umeboshi vinegar to taste. Toss gently and serve.

Sautéed Kale

We eat so much kale in our family, so I try to mix it up a bit, alternating between the steamed recipe and this sautéed version. If the rest of the food we're having at a meal is lightly flavored, I make this kale, because it has more seasoning.

Serves 4

Ingredients
- 1 bunch kale (1 pound), torn into bite-size pieces
- 1 tablespoon extra-virgin olive oil
- 2 teaspoons soy sauce
- 1 garlic clove, put through a garlic press

1. Heat a medium-size skillet over low heat. Add the oil, soy sauce, and garlic. Stir until the garlic turns golden.
2. Add the kale and continue cooking, stirring continuously, for 3 minutes.

Broiled Asparagus

These are like healthy French fries, because placing asparagus in a broiler makes them crispy at the edges.

Serves 4

Ingredients
1 bunch asparagus (1 pound)
1 tablespoon extra-virgin olive oil
1 ½ tablespoons fresh lemon juice (about ½ lemon)
⅛ teaspoon Sea Veg

1. Cut off 1 inch of asparagus stems on the diagonal, soak in salt water for 5 minutes, and rinse well. Place asparagus in a steamer basket inside a large pot. Add 1 cup water. Bring to a boil. Steam for 3 minutes.
2. While asparagus are steaming, turn oven to broil setting.
3. When asparagus are bright green and tender, place on cookie sheet, in a single layer. Drizzle with oil and lemon juice, and sprinkle with Sea Veg.
4. Place seasoned asparagus under broiler for 1 to 2 minutes, tops, until crispy.

Sweet Carrots

Arianna really likes these carrots, and Addison will eat them if they're really sweet. You can serve them in chunks, as I do, or mash them up into "carrot mash." With a sweet dish like this, I'm the one who tastes it to see if it has enough agave, not my children—or else there'd be half a bottle in there.

Serves 4

Ingredients

    1 bunch carrots (½ pound, preferably organic), cut into 1-inch pieces
    Agave to taste
    Cinnamon to taste

1. Place carrots in a pot with enough water to cover them, plus two inches. Cover.
2. Bring to a boil and cook for 7 to 10 minutes, until carrots are soft enough that a fork slides easily into them.
3. Drain the carrots and return them to the pot. Add agave and cinnamon and serve.

Roasted Brussels Sprouts

These are a favorite of mine, and I'm happy to say that Arianna likes them, too. (Addison's not there yet, but I'm hopeful.)

Serves 4

Ingredients
   1 pound Brussels sprouts (1 round container in most markets)
   1 tablespoon extra-virgin olive oil
   2 teaspoons balsamic vinegar
   ½ teaspoon Sea Veg

1. Preheat oven to 375°F.
2. Trim stem ends of Brussels sprouts and cut in half.
3. Pour 2 cups water into a medium pot with a steamer basket. Add Brussels sprouts and steam for 3 to 5 minutes, until tender to the core.
4. Drizzle the oil on a cookie sheet. Add 1 teaspoon balsamic vinegar and ¼ teaspoon Sea Veg. Blend by hand to coat pan evenly.
5. Place steamed Brussels sprouts, cut side down, on the cookie sheet and drizzle them with remaining vinegar and Sea Veg.
6. Place cookie sheet in the oven for 10 to 12 minutes, until Brussels sprouts are crisp at the edges. For extra-crispy ones, put the oven on broil for the last minute.

Pureed Carrots for Baby

I made these carrots for both my kids when they were babies. No one I personally knew at the time was making fresh, homemade, organic baby food, and my mother teased me about starting my own baby food company. Because this dish doesn't contain any preservatives, it lasts just two days in the fridge. After that, chuck it.

Makes 1 ½ cups

Ingredients

5 small carrots (preferably organic), peeled and cut into ½-inch pieces

1. Put carrots in a pot with enough water to cover plus 1 inch. Bring to a boil.
2. Cook for 7 to 10 minutes, until soft enough that a fork slides into them easily.
3. Scoop carrots out with a slotted spoon and place in a blender with ½ cup of the cooking water. Puree.

My Sisters' Cucumbers

My two sisters and I grew up eating these cucumbers. It was one of the few things we could make when our mother wasn't home. Today, Arianna loves them as a side with lunch or dinner, or a snack

Serves 4

Ingredients

2 cucumbers, peeled and cut into ¼-inch rounds or long, thin strips
¼ cup raw apple cider vinegar
⅓ cup water
½ teaspoon Sea Veg

Place cucumbers in a bowl. Add the vinegar, water, and Sea Veg. Toss well and let sit for 15 minutes, or chill until ready to serve.

SOUPS AND RICE

Carrot Ginger Soup

This can be an appetizer or a light meal. For a thinner consistency, add additional cooking liquid.

Serves 4

Ingredients
14 carrots, peeled and cut into 1-inch pieces
2 tablespoons peeled and grated ginger (3-inch piece of ginger)

1. Put carrots in a medium-size pot with enough water to cover plus 2 inches.
2. Bring to a boil and cook for 10 minutes, or until carrots are easily pierced with a fork.
3. Scoop carrots out of the pot with a slotted spoon and place in a blender.
4. Add 1 ¾ cups of the cooking water. Blend until smooth and creamy. Add additional liquid for a thinner consistency.
5. Squeeze the ginger pulp with a garlic press over a small bowl. It will yield about 1 to 2 teaspoons juice. Discard pulp. Add ginger juice into creamy carrots to taste, and stir.

Miso Soup

Miso has beneficial bacteria and healing properties. It's something we've been eating since Mina came into our lives. (Back then, she had us eating it for breakfast.) Just make sure you add the miso after you've cooked all the other ingredients, since miso that's cooked loses its nutrients. Also, if you heat the soup up the next day, add a little bit of fresh miso to get all the benefits.

Serves 4

Ingredients

5 cups water
1-inch piece kombu, broken up
1-inch piece wakame, broken up
¼ pound firm tofu, finely diced
1 tablespoon adzuki bean miso (optional varieties are barley or rice)
1 teaspoon scallions, finely sliced

1. Combine the water, kombu, wakame, and tofu in a medium pot. Gently bring to a boil. Reduce the heat and simmer for 10 minutes.
2. Turn the heat off. Place miso into a small bowl and ladle ¼ cup of the hot liquid into it. Stir until miso paste is dissolved. Add mixture back into the pot. Stir in scallions and serve.

Broccoli Soup

Serves 4

Ingredients
1 bunch broccoli
Sea Veg to taste

1. Cut off bottom inch of broccoli stem. Chop the florets and remaining stems coarsely. Put broccoli in a medium pot and add enough water to cover plus two inches. Bring to a boil covered.
2. Cook 10 minutes or until a fork pierces the broccoli easily.
3. Scoop broccoli with a slotted spoon directly into a blender.
4. Add 1 ½ cups of the cooking water and blend until creamy.
5. Season with Sea Veg to taste.

Kombu Rice

I use kombu in my rice. This Japanese seaweed provides many vitamins and minerals that are hard to get from other foods. You can leave the kombu in when you serve the rice or take it out. Either way, by cooking them together your rice gets infused with some of the kombu's nutrients. You can also make this dish using quinoa rather than rice.

Serves 4

Ingredients
   1 cup white jasmine or short-grain brown rice
   1-inch piece kombu

1. Soak rice for 30 minutes in a bowl with cool water. Drain and rinse with fresh water.
2. Place rice in a pot with 1 ½ cups water. (For brown rice, use 2 cups water.)
3. Add kombu and cover with a lid. Bring to a boil. Lower heat, and simmer, lid halfway on, 10 to 15 minutes. (For brown rice, cook 45 minutes.)
4. Remove pot from heat and let rice sit for 5 minutes. Fluff with a fork and serve.

BEANS

Mom's Lentils with Kale

This is a doctored version of my mom's lentil recipe, one she made when I was growing up. Once I discovered sea vegetables and umeboshi, I tweaked the recipe a bit. You can put these lentils on top of rice or eat them alone. The leftovers can become a soup the next day if you add about ⅓ cup water when heating them up.

Serves 4 to 6

Ingredients

1 ½ cups dried French lentils
2-inch piece of kombu
1 carrot, cut into ½-inch pieces
1 stalk of celery, cut into ½-inch pieces
½ teaspoon cumin
1 teaspoon curry
1 teaspoon garlic powder
½ teaspoon Sea Veg
2 cups bite-size pieces kale, stems removed
2 teaspoons umeboshi vinegar

1. Sort through the lentils, removing any pebbles. Rinse in water. Soak in 2 ½ cups water for 4 hours. (I've done this even when the bag says eight hours, and it works.)
2. Strain lentils and add to a medium-size pot with 5 cups water and drop in a piece of kombu. Bring to a boil. Lower flame to a simmer. Skim and discard any foam that rises to the top. Cover and cook 40 minutes.
3. Add the carrot, celery, cumin, curry, and garlic powder. Cook another 15 to 20 minutes with the lid off.
4. Add the kale and vinegar. Cook 5 to 10 more minutes.

Adzuki Beans

Mina Dobic introduced me to adzuki beans (also spelled azuki), and I've been making them ever since. They're low in fat and sodium and high in protein, fiber, complex carbohydrates, iron, and potassium. They are believed to benefit the bladder, reproductive function, and kidneys; help prevent breast cancer; provide a good source of energy; promote regular bowel function; lower cholesterol; and tone the lungs. I make a pot of them at the beginning of the week, and they become the core of our dinners for a few nights. The first night, I'll serve them with white jasmine rice or steamed kale. The next night, I'll serve them with tofu and kale or rice. The third night, I may spread the beans on a tortilla with rice and melt or sprinkle dairy-free cheese on top.

Serves 4

Ingredients
1 cup dried adzuki beans
1-inch piece wakame
1-inch piece kombu
½ teaspoon umeboshi vinegar
¼ teaspoon Sea Veg
1 teaspoon adzuki bean miso

1. Sort through the beans, removing any pebbles. Rinse beans. Place in a bowl with 3 cups water and soak overnight.
2. Strain the beans and place in a medium-size pot with 3 cups water, the wakame, and the kombu.
3. Bring to a boil. Lower heat and cook, covered, until beans are soft, not mushy, 40 to 50 minutes. Stir several times during cooking.
4. When beans are tender, add the umeboshi, Sea Veg, and adzuki bean miso. Stir well to combine.

Black Beans

Beans are a staple in my home because they're so versatile. You can use them as part of a meal with other sides, such as tofu or kale. You can also mash them up and make a bean dip. It's a great way to get all the nutrients of beans and add variety to your meals. I make a pot of these one day, doubling the recipe, and use them throughout the week. In fact, they taste better the second day because they've had a chance to marinate in their seasonings.

Serves 4

Ingredients

1 cup dried black beans
1-inch piece wakame
1-inch piece kombu
½ cup fresh cilantro, coarsely chopped (or 1 tablespoon dried)
4 garlic cloves, put through a garlic press
1 tablespoon fresh-squeezed lemon juice (about ½ lemon)
3 tablespoons fresh-squeezed lime juice (about 1 lime)
½ teaspoon Sea Veg
½ teaspoon umeboshi vinegar

1. Sort through the beans, removing any pebbles. Rinse the beans and place in a bowl with 3 cups water. Soak overnight.
2. Drain the beans and place in a medium-size pot with 3 to 4 cups water. (If you want a bean stew, add less water; for a soup, add more.)
3. Add the wakame, kombu, cilantro, and garlic. Bring to a boil. Lower heat and cook, with the lid slightly ajar, 1 hour and 15 minutes, stirring several times.
4. When beans are soft and creamy, add the lemon juice, lime juice, umeboshi vinegar, and Sea Veg. Stir well and turn off heat.

Bean Tortillas

This is a great way to combine leftover beans into a fresh, new meal or a snack. These tortillas are delicious with a side of steamed kale or broccoli, or roasted asparagus.

Makes 4 tortillas

Ingredients

    1 teaspoon extra-virgin olive oil
    Four 6-inch corn tortillas
    2 cups cooked black or adzuki beans (see Black Beans recipe)
    1 cup cooked brown rice
    1 cup shredded, dairy-free white and/or yellow cheese
    1 lime cut into 4 wedges

1. Heat a small skillet over medium heat. Add the oil.
2. Place 1 tortilla into the pan and cook for 1 minute. Flip over and cook another minute. Repeat with remaining tortillas.
3. Layer each tortilla with ½ cup beans, ¼ cup rice, and top with ¼ cup cheese. Squeeze a wedge of lime on tortilla just before eating.

Hummus

Arianna loves to eat this hummus warm with crackers, cucumbers, carrots, or olives. It's a great snack or side dish with dinner. Serve it chilled or at room temperature. You can also put it on a turkey sandwich as a healthier alternative to mayonnaise, or make a vegetarian sandwich with hummus, avocado, and some great bread or a tortilla shell.

Serves 4

Ingredients
   1 ½ cups dried garbanzo beans (aka chickpeas)
   2 tablespoons extra-virgin olive oil
   ¾ teaspoon sea salt
   3 tablespoons fresh lemon juice (about 1 lemon)
   ½ teaspoon umeboshi vinegar

1. Sort through beans, removing pebbles. Rinse beans and place in a bowl with 3 ½ cups water. Soak overnight.
2. Drain the beans and put into a medium-size pot. Add 5 cups water. Bring to a boil. Lower heat and cook, covered, for 1 ½ hours or until beans are very tender.
3. Scoop chickpeas out with a slotted spoon and into a food processor or blender. Add ½ cup of the chickpea cooking liquid. Puree until smooth. Add the oil, sea salt, lemon juice, and umeboshi vinegar. Let sit at room temperature, to cool, before serving.

QUICK DISHES

Kale Chips

These chips are perfect for when you're craving something salty, but healthy. The kale should be crispy after at least 20 minutes of cooking time. If it's soggy, you probably used too much olive oil.

Makes 3 cups of chips

Ingredients
1 bunch kale (one pound)
1 tablespoon extra-virgin olive oil
¼ teaspoon Sea Veg
1 ½ tablespoons fresh lemon juice (about ½ lemon)

1. Preheat oven to 350°F.
2. Remove stems from kale and tear leaves into big pieces. Soak in cold water with 1 tablespoon sea salt. Rinse well.
3. Strain kale and pat dry with paper towels to blot excess water.
4. Drizzle oil and Sea Veg on a cookie sheet lined with parchment paper. Add kale and toss with oil and salt. (It may seem like a lot of greens, but kale shrinks by half as it cooks.)
5. Place cookie sheet in the oven. Bake for 10 minutes. Sprinkle lemon juice on top of kale. Toss like a salad on the tray. Place back into the oven for another 10 minutes.
6. Bake for a total of 20 to 25 minutes. Kale is done when it's crispy.

Mashed Sweet Potatoes

Sweet potatoes aren't just for Thanksgiving. We eat them often. They give you the nutrients you need and can satisfy a sweet tooth at the same time.

Serves 4

Ingredients

2 large sweet potatoes or yams (2 pounds), washed, peeled, and cut into 1-inch pieces

2 teaspoons Earth Balance butter (available at health food stores)

½ teaspoon cinnamon

1 tablespoon agave, or to taste

Sea salt to taste

1. Put sweet potatoes into a medium-size pot and add enough cold water to cover by 1 inch.
2. Bring to a boil and cook for 15 to 20 minutes, or until a fork pierces the potato easily.
3. Drain the potatoes in a colander. Return them to the pot. Add butter, cinnamon, agave, and sea salt. Mash until smooth.

Daddy's Sunday Sandwich

My husband's schedule is full, so he doesn't cook much, but on weekends he likes to experiment in the kitchen, which is how this sandwich was created. My kids love it so much they told me, "Please put this in your book!" It's a great lunch or after-school snack.

Ingredients

    3 slices turkey lunch meat
    1 teaspoon extra-virgin olive oil
    3 slices turkey bacon
    Wheat bread (we use bread Addison can eat, but any kind works)
    Coarse black pepper to taste
    Vegenaise or mustard (optional)

1. Heat a skillet for 2 minutes. Add the oil and the turkey bacon. Cook according to package directions.
2. When bacon is done, drain on paper towels and set aside. In the same hot skillet, place the slices of turkey lunch meat for 30 seconds. Flip them over and heat for another 30 seconds. (You're just warming it up, not actually cooking it.)
3. Warm the bread up in the toaster (don't toast it).
4. Place turkey bacon, turkey meat, and a sprinkle of coarse black pepper on one piece of bread. Top that with another slice of bread. Add condiments, if using.

Brown Rice Pasta with Marinara

I don't always cook meals from scratch. You can make healthy meals by doctoring up store-bought products. Here's a perfect example. It's a meal I make when I need something delicious and satisfying but don't have a lot of time. The brown rice pasta is a good complex carb without any white flour, and adding fresh ingredients to the jarred sauce makes it come alive. I serve it with a side of steamed broccoli with flaxseed oil and I've got a meal in fifteen minutes, tops!

Serves 4

Ingredients

   2 tablespoons extra-virgin olive oil
   12-ounce package of brown rice pasta, any shape
   16-ounce jar organic marinara sauce
   5 fresh basil leaves, torn into small pieces
   ¼ teaspoon dried basil
   1 teaspoon lemon juice
   ½ teaspoon soy sauce
   ⅛ teaspoon Sea Veg
   2 small garlic cloves, minced

1. Combine 8 cups water with oil in a medium-size pot and bring to a boil.
2. Add pasta. Cook for 10 to 12 minutes, stirring several times.
3. While pasta is cooking, pour sauce into a small pot. Add fresh basil, dried basil, lemon juice, soy sauce, Sea Veg, and minced garlic. Simmer 5 to 10 minutes.
4. When the pasta is tender, strain and rinse with cool, not cold, water.
5. Place pasta in a serving bowl and add the sauce. Mix well and serve.

Tofu Scramble

Depending on my mood, I may add a squeeze of lemon juice after I finish cooking this. Arianna will eat it if I add some cheese. It can also be served on top of gluten-free, wheat-free bread. Try a sprinkle of flaxseed or ground flax meal on top.

Serves 2

Ingredients

2 teaspoons extra-virgin olive oil

1 tablespoon plus 1 teaspoon soy sauce

¼ teaspoon Sea Veg

14-ounce package extra-firm tofu, rinsed and drained on a paper towel

½ teaspoon curry powder

¼ teaspoon turmeric

1 ½ tablespoons fresh-squeezed lemon juice (about ½ lemon)

1. Heat the oil in a small skillet on medium heat.
2. Add the soy sauce and Sea Veg. Crumble the tofu into the pan.
3. Add the curry powder and turmeric. Stir as if scrambling eggs for 3 minutes. Pour the lemon juice over the tofu, mix, and serve.

BREAKFASTS

Smooth Smoothies

Vary your smoothie ingredients depending on your taste. For example, if you want it to be a pretty red color, add more raspberries. When we have leftover smoothie mix I make ice pops by pouring the mix into an ice pop maker (ordered online from Amazon) or an ice cube tray. If you use an ice cube tray, lay a piece of foil on top after pouring the mixture into the tray and then put wooden ice pop sticks (available online at Amazon or Market America) through the foil.

Makes four ½-cup servings

Ingredients
- 1 cup of R.W. Knudsen organic apple juice
- 1 cup blueberries
- 1 cup raspberries
- 1 cup sliced strawberries
- 1 banana (optional, as thickener; or use ½ to ¾ cup juice)

1. Place all ingredients in a blender. Blend until very smooth, 30 to 40 seconds. Pour into glasses and serve.

Crunchy Oatmeal

I make this recipe daily during the school year because it takes no time and can be tweaked according to taste. The options for toppings are endless, but some suggestions include fresh apricots, banana slices, and maple syrup.

Serves 4

Ingredients

2 cups rolled oats (gluten-free, but you can use any kind)
½ cup raisins
¼ teaspoon cinnamon
1 tablespoon agave
1 cup blueberries or raspberries
1 cup granola

1. Combine oats and 4 cups water in a medium-size pot. Mix. Bring to a boil. Lower heat and cook, covered, for 10 minutes, stirring occasionally, until creamy.
2. Take off the stove and add raisins, cinnamon, and agave. Top each bowl with ¼ cup berries and ¼ cup granola.

Homemade Mochi Waffles

These dairy-free, egg-free, wheat-free waffles are a big hit with my kids and their friends. Addison likes them with mixed berry yogurt. You can also sprinkle them with flaxseed. We make this as a dessert, too, by adding rice or soy ice cream and chocolate syrup.

Makes 4 waffles

Ingredients

Coconut oil or olive oil (I prefer coconut oil because it gives you extra nutrients)

12 ½–ounce package mochi, shredded on a box grater or cut into 4 equal pieces (available at health food stores, in the refrigerated section)

Agave (or maple syrup) to taste

1. Preheat your waffle maker on 4 or a higher setting.
2. Brush oil on the waffle iron and add ¾ cup shredded mochi or 1 square to waffle iron.
3. Cook for 5 minutes or until well melted. Repeat with rest of mochi. Top each waffle with agave or maple syrup, fresh fruit or eat plain.

Cheese Melt Bagel

This is great for breakfast, lunch, or a yummy, cheesy snack. I use soy cheese because of Addison's allergies, but regular cream cheese and cheddar cheese will work, too. We also opt for spelt bagels, but traditional ones work fine.

Makes 2 bagels

Ingredients
Soy cream cheese
2 bagels, sliced in half
4 slices soy yellow cheddar cheese

1. Spread soy cream cheese on each half of the bagel.
2. Top each half with one slice of cheese.
3. Place in broiler for one minute, until cheese is completely melted.

Cinnamon Agave Toast

This is a quick, easy breakfast that Arianna loves.

Makes 2 pieces toast

Ingredients

1 ½ teaspoons Earth Balance butter
2 slices spelt or traditional bread
2 teaspoons agave
¼ teaspoon cinnamon
1 teaspoon ground flaxseed (optional)

1. Spread the butter on side of the bread that is face side up.
2. Mix the agave and cinnamon in a small bowl. Spread the mixture on each slice.
3. Put the bread under the broiler for 45 seconds, until it's a little crispy on the edges.
4. Remove. If desired, sprinkle ground flaxseed on each slice.

SWEETS

Oatmeal-Raisin Cookies

My kids love these for dessert, but they're also great for school bake sales. They're quick, easy, and healthy.

Makes 24 cookies

Ingredients
2 cups oatmeal
½ cup raisins
1 ½ teaspoons cinnamon
3 tablespoons spelt flour
½ cup maple syrup
¼ cup agave
1 cup applesauce (homemade or store bought)
¾ teaspoon vanilla extract
1 tablespoon refined coconut oil

1. Preheat oven to 350°F.
2. Combine ingredients and mix until well blended.
3. Scoop mixture by tablespoon onto a cookie sheet lined with parchment paper, placed 1 inch apart. Flatten a little bit with your finger or the back of a spoon.
4. Bake for 25 minutes, until golden brown.

Dairy-Free Banana Split

This is a great way to enjoy ice cream that's dairy-free and delicious. Addison loves this one.

Serves 2

Ingredients
   1 banana sliced in half lengthwise
   3 scoops soy or rice vanilla ice cream
   Dairy-free, gluten-free chocolate syrup
   Soy or rice whipped cream (found in dairy section of health food store)

1. Divide banana halves between two bowls.
2. Top with ice cream.
3. Drizzle with chocolate syrup and whipped cream.

Arianna and Addison's Rice Crispy Treats

I've been making these treats for years now, and my kids love them. Addison often brings them to school with his lunch. Sometimes I add dried blueberries, dried raspberries, or vegan chocolate chips. If you want thicker treats, use a smaller glass baking dish. For thinner ones, use a larger dish.

Makes eighteen 3-inch squares

Ingredients
10-ounce Rice Twice Gluten Free Cereal (Erewhon)
Two 10-ounce containers Suzanne's Ricemellow Creme (dairy-free; found in baking section of health food store or ordered online)
3 ½ tablespoons Earth Balance butter
1 teaspoon vanilla extract
Olive oil to coat glass baking dish

1. Heat Suzanne's Ricemellow Creme in a large pot on low to medium heat.
2. Add the butter, stirring with a rubber spatula for 5 minutes, until soft and melted together.
3. Add the vanilla. Pour 1 cup of cereal at a time into the hot pot, mixing, until the entire box is used. Mix well to combine. Cook for 5 minutes.
4. Pour mixture into a lightly oiled, 9-by-13-inch glass baking dish. Smooth and level with the spatula.
5. Set aside for 30 minutes to cool and firm up. Cut into eighteen 3-inch squares.

Kanten

I learned how to make kanten the year we went macrobiotic, and my kids still love this dessert today. It's a healthy version of Jell-O that's so easy to prepare. You can cut it into cake-size squares or blend it until it's creamy. Add some fresh lemon juice. My kids love it both ways!

Serves 4

Ingredients
   4 tablespoons agar flakes
   1 quart juice (I like pomegranate-blueberry blend)
   ½ lemon (optional)

1. Combine agar flakes and juice in a medium pot. Stir together and gently bring to a boil, about 5 minutes.
2. Reduce heat and simmer for 10 minutes, stirring several times, until flakes are dissolved.
3. Pour mixture into a 10-inch-square glass baking dish. Let dish sit at room temperature to cool, until there is no steam rising. Place in refrigerator for 1 hour or until firm to the touch. Cut into desired-size pieces, or blend until creamy, and add lemon juice.

Easy Applesauce

My family eats this applesauce for a snack or dessert. It's also great for babies. You can spread it on rice cakes, add a spoonful to your oatmeal, or eat it plain. I like to sprinkle cinnamon on top just before serving, in case someone doesn't like cinnamon. To give it a pretty color, you can blend in raspberries. It keeps for 2 days in the refrigerator.

Makes 4 cups

Ingredients

8 Gala or Red Delicious apples (preferably organic), peeled and cut into 2-inch pieces
1 pint raspberries (optional)
Dash of cinnamon

1. Place apples in a medium-size pot with 2 cups cold water. Cover and bring to a boil. Cook for 10 minutes, or until apples can be pierced easily with a fork.
2. Remove half of the apples with a slotted spoon and place directly in a blender. (If using berries, add them now.) Blend until pureed. (Reserve ¼ cup cooking liquid for blending, if you need it.) Pour into a serving bowl. Repeat with remaining cooked apples.
3. Set applesauce aside to cool. Sprinkle cinnamon lightly on top of individual servings, if desired.

BEVERAGES

Chuck-the-Soda Soda

At a restaurant, I'll let my kids have a Shirley Temple or ginger ale, but if they want a sweet, fizzy drink at home, we make this version of soda. My kids love the lime and lemon, and I'd rather have them drink this than Sprite. After all, it's served in a glass, not in aluminum, and we add our own sweetener.

Makes 2 drinks

Ingredients

    2 cups club soda or sparkling water
    Juice of either 1 lime, lemon, or orange
    2 teaspoons agave (optional)

1. Pour club soda or sparkling water into 2 glasses.
2. Divide the juice of your choice between the two glasses.
3. Add 1 teaspoon agave to each glass, if using. Stir and enjoy.

Sparkling Cranberry Fizz

Here's another way to enjoy a fruity, fizzy drink that's not too sweet.

Serves 2

Ingredients

2 cups club soda

⅔ cup sweetened cranberry juice or unsweetened apple juice

1. Pour club soda into 2 glasses.
2. Divide the juice between the two glasses. Stir and enjoy.

The Rona

This drink is named after a friend of mine who is macrobiotic. She drank it every morning when she came to visit us last summer, and got me hooked on it. Now I have it every morning, too. You'll need a juicer for this one.

Makes 4 cups

Ingredients

    3 cucumbers, peeled and cut in half lengthwise
    4-inch piece daikon root, cut in half lengthwise
    2 lemons, quartered (organic, if possible)
    5 celery stalks
    3 kale leaves

1. Put the cucumbers, daikon, lemon, celery, and kale, one at a time, through a juicer. Stir the fresh juice, pour into glasses, and drink immediately.

Soothing Tea with Manuka

Manuka honey, which comes from New Zealand, is known for its concentrated and unique healing properties. This is a drink I give my kids when they have a sore throat or want to warm up on a cold day.

Serves 2

Ingredients

Fresh-squeezed lemon juice (½ lemon)
1 teaspoon manuka honey (available at health food stores)

1. Boil 2 cups water. Turn off heat.
2. Add the lemon juice and honey.
3. Stir well, pour into cups, and drink hot.

HEALING WITH FOOD

Here are some simple, healing foods:

MANUKA HONEY FOR A SORE THROAT OR COUGH: If my kids' throats hurt or if they have a cough, I give them a spoonful of this honey from New Zealand known for its healing properties. (A little bit of manuka honey is also great on a rice cake or as a sweet snack, especially when you're trying to wean your kids off sugar.)

APPLE CIDER VINEGAR FOR A SORE THROAT: I warm ½ cup of apple cider vinegar on the stove. Then I add ½ teaspoon sea salt, stir it together, and have my kids gargle with it until it's gone. I also give them each 1 teaspoon of apple cider vinegar to take. This is great to do when strep throat is going around. Apple cider vinegar is known for its healing benefits related to certain health conditions, such as sore throats and weight loss.

WHITE ONION FOR AN EARACHE: Cut a nice, round slice of a white onion, a big enough piece to cover the ear. Place it in a steamer basket or a two-pot steamer with water for 2 to 3 minutes, until it is slightly soft and changes color a little bit. (You don't want to cook it too long or you'll lose some of the nutrients.) Place the entire onion slice—and all its layers—on top of the ear that hurts (it's fine if onion juice gets in the ear). On top of this, place a warm, moist paper towel and a hot water bottle or a warm washcloth. Hold in place for 20 to 30 minutes. Repeat twice a day.

PEPPERMINT TEA FOR A FEVER: I boil water and steep four peppermint tea bags in a pot. I have my kids take a lukewarm bath and while they're in the tub, I dip a washcloth into the pot of peppermint tea and sponge under their armpits, on the backs of their necks, and on their heads. (Think of a sponge bath with peppermint tea.) When they get out of the tub, I have them dress in warm clothes—sweatpants, long-sleeve shirts, socks—and drink something warm, such as the manuka honey tea, before they get into bed. In the middle of the night, they have to change their clothes because they're sweating so much, but this is the point, since the tea helps draw their fever out.

Alternative Birthday Party Menu

My kids have gone to countless birthday parties in the last few years, and I'm always amazed at the food that is served: take-out pizza or chicken nuggets. It would be fine if this were a once-in-a-while thing, but if your kids are like mine, it seems there's a birthday party every other weekend.

An alternative birthday menu could include the following recipes, which are all quick, easy, and a big hit with kids: Chicken Strips, quesadillas (with chicken or cheese), Broiled Asparagus (which are crisp like French fries), or Steamed Broccoli. Then have some sliced fruit or applesauce and serve the Sparkling Cranberry Fizz drink (or just sparkling water in a glass with a slice of lemon on the side to look festive). Top that off with your cake or cupcakes. This way you'll still enjoy a fun, festive party with a sweet treat!

Products Mentioned

Benadryl
CARES (Child Aviation Restraint System): www.kidsflysafe.com
Dr. Bronner's Magic Soaps
EpiPen
Klean Kanteen water bottle: www.kleankanteen.com
Niosh Mask N95
Sea Veg: www.seaveg.com/shop/index.php?main_page=page&id=22
Seventh Generation dishwasher soap
Sigg water bottle: www.mysigg.com
Washington Homeopathic Products: www.homeopathyworks.com/jshop/section
.php?xSec=51&jssCart=3b45ea7c0bef928eba3b00622ccae8d5

Acknowledgments

My best friend—I thank you God for believing in me, for using me and making me the vessel used to utilize this information you put on my journey and to share with those in the world. Having you in my life is the *only* reason this is even possible. I thank you, and I love you deeply.

Baby, wow, look at little Erica, your gypsy wife. Thank you for asking for my hand in marriage to be your wife. Aside from you always making sure I am the queen in the palace, and giving me your love and support, the most irreplaceable and priceless gift of them all is the gift of your two children we created together. With us, there is Arianna and Addison—*Je t'aime*.

To my children from my core: Arianna, my lovely daughter, you have brought me sunshine from the second you were born. As my firstborn, you were my first teacher when I became your mother, and I thank God for you *every day*. With you, this book was born. Thank you. You are so full of compassion, love, determination, will, strength, fire, and much more. Because of you, I push to achieve more. I try to lead by example. You were the one taking pictures of Mommy signing contracts for this book, jumping up and down with me and sharing my excitement. Always ready to cheer me on as my biggest cheerleader. Thank you. I admire how brave and persistent you are. You make me so proud of who you are and who you are becoming. You have your own journey to walk; therefore, follow yours and know that I am your biggest cheerleader. Stay on your own path, please be yourself, and let your inner voice be the first voice you listen to. Know that passion can be discovered at any age as you have taught me. *Your* happiness is *in you*. Always remain positive, in balance, true to yourself, and take care of your biggest blessing—you.

I love being your mommy. I love you no matter what. Thank you for being my daughter. Love forever, your Mommy.

Addison, my loving, handsome son, you are a gift in itself. I thank God for giving you to me to borrow, to learn with, to learn from, and to be enlightened by your spirit and your awareness. I am so thankful for all that we have experienced together as mother and son. I thought I was done learning about being a mommy, until I had you. The health challenges you were given were a blessing, because we were able to give life to this book and help you and many others. Together we learned that many things are possible if we just *believe*. Embrace all of who *you* are and accept *everything* about you. I am so proud of you and how you respect yourself and care for Addison. I *love* the person you *are* and who you are becoming, and I accept *everything* about you. Always continue to take care of yourself and your health, and *never* be afraid to speak up by using the voice you were given. Focus on the positivity of life. We only see change by making change, so be the change you want to change! Follow your dreams and know that I support them. We did this book with your help and your push, thank you. I love you more than you will ever know. Love Addison and look inside of Addison and sit still for your guidance. Your answers will *always* come in silence. Thank you for being you. Thank you for being my son. I love being your mom. I love you no matter what. Love forever, your Mommy.

My children from my heart: Tony, Aaron, and Ashley, *no* matter what, *always* know that I love each of you. Be who God put you here to be. Follow your own dreams and *achieve* them. Be only who you are to be. You cannot buy happiness, but you can create it. I love you.

My parents: Mom, you have always been the first woman I idolized and looked up to. Always put together, beautiful, smelling good, and so nurturing to your daughters. Thank you for the wonderful life you gave to me, thank you for my sisters. Thank you for the fond childhood memories that were so special. You being a single parent most of my life, I now know what it took and what you gave to make it all possible. I thank you for never losing your sanity and for allowing me to spread my wings to experience the world outside of ours. I love life and it has so much to do with my yesterdays that you provided. Mom, thank you for everything. Thank you for sharing yourself and being a wonderful mother. Thank you for all the sacrifices you made on my behalf. I love you *forever* and I am still fond of you and so thankful for you. Your Volvo is never forgotten. Love always, your second daughter.

Daddy, life presents us with things for a reason, as you know. I thank you for being in my life today and being a great grandfather to my babies. Yesterday does not matter, today does. Thank you for your love and for the fun days we continue to have. I love you.

Brigette, achieve all you desire. Nothing ever gets in our way except ourselves! Know that I love you, I am always here for you, proud of you, and so thankful to have you as my sister. I *love* you forever.

Angela, my sister and my closest friend, *always* there for me *no* matter what! Twins, but not. I know you are laughing right now at the fact that I did a book and made it out of college with a degree. I am always here for you and I thank you for everything, especially for babysitting. I love you dearly.

Gabrielle, I love you. You are so caring and truly special. Embrace how God made you and love everything about yourself. The day you came into my life, I felt my heart. Thank you for being in my life. I love you.

Dearest Nana, you are the rock and the glue for our family. You made all things possible for each and every one of us. I am so grateful to you and all you have ever done for me. I love you more than I show. Nana, thank you for sharing everything you had with me, especially my mother. Nana, I love you more.

Dear Grandma Holton, thank you for all those kosher pickles and sweet potato pies. Thank you for my Dad. I love you.

Ms. Reid, thank you for your son and for always coming to visit. I love you.

Aunt Carol, thank you for all your belief, faith, and trust in me to complete this project. You were right on the sidelines screaming me on and your voice was what I needed. Thank you for caring. I love you dearly.

Jack, Chris, Quentin, Liberty, Taylor, and all your children: I am glad we are family. I love you all. Dream high. If you really want it, *go get it*!

Grandaddy, I love and miss you. You started this book, and I finished it.

Marsha, my loving *godmother,* I miss you dearly—love you.

Bliss, I love and miss you.

Aunt Mert, I think of you often. I miss you, and I thank you. I love you.

Aerian, I miss you more than ever. Thank you for teaching me how to take care of your siblings. I am so proud of who you became—I love you.

Janis, thank you for being in our lives, and for showing me the good life, speaking French, and how to handle a taxi driver in the Big Apple. xo.

Nik'ki Hennings, you are the definition of *supermom*, and truly an *incredible* mother—nine kids and you have kept your sanity, your natural looks, and your spirit. *You* are the one I learned so much from, how to be an involved and really hands-on mom. Thank you for entrusting me with your children, and for sharing them with me. You are so special and one who deserves only days full of sunshine. I love you all.

Crystal Crystal Crystal, all because of a simple conversation you and I had one summer at my table, this ball got rolling. Thank you, and thank you for Lisa, and thank you for all your continuous support, friendship, and for sharing your knowledge. Big hug.

To all my dear friends, you each know who you are and I thank you all from deep in my heart for allowing me to laugh, cry, disconnect to write this book, for your nonstop support, and most of all, for always being there for me no matter what. Thank you for being a real friend to me. I love you and I cherish what I have with each of you.

Ariella, you are a huge constant help and so amazing. I truly appreciate you. Thank you for sharing your love.

Catherine, thank you for being so sweet, loving, and there! xo. Diana—so dedicated—*muchas gracias por todo*. Belkis, you are incredible. Thank you, thank you, thank you. Lissette, thank you for all you do. Zulma, I still need you; you are truly missed. Yasmine. thank you for being born.

To the lovely girls who allow me to mentor them: Krystal, Tiranke, Tyanah, Awa, Hawa, and Abigail. You each are special in your own way and I am *very* proud of you girls. *Please* aim *high* for yourselves. Never settle. Respect and love yourself *first*. Thank you for sharing your life with me. You all make me smile and I love our time together. Be positive, read, and explore to make yourself knowledgeable, embrace your experiences, and learn from your mistakes as they are our life lessons. Love, Ms. Erica.

Book contributors: Thank you to all the contributors and experts who shared a quote, shared their expertise, their patience, their time, their efforts, their perspective, their opinion, their knowledge, and themselves. Margie Sherard, Pattie Mallette, Nicole Richie, Lori Stokes, Dr. Barbara Landreth,

Ricki Lake, Laila Ali, Dr. Fred Pescatore, Bobbi Brown, Malaak Compton-Rock, Melissa Etheridge, Gayle King, Sara Keagle, Marianne Williamson, Jeffrey May, Veronica Webb, Stefanie Sacks, Holly Robinson Peete, and Jan Schlossberg. Each and every one of you contributed in a big way and I am always grateful for it. Thank you for being available to do this and for saying yes and coming through. Thank you, thank you, thank you—you all are *amazing* and added special ingredients to this book! I share this with you *all*! *Thank you* from deep down in my heart.

Majid Ali, Mina Dobic, the world needs to know more about you both. Thank you for sharing your knowledge, your wisdom, and for healing my conditions along with my children's. You both are *huge blessings*.

Thank you to Simone, Gabriel, Dr. Asher, Dr. Barbara, Dr. Pescatore, Dr. Manos, Dr. Bayno, Dr. Lipman, Ora Abel-Russel, Damien, our doula, Nathalie, Ivonne, Ms. So, Rachel, and anyone else who has aided in the healing of my children and myself. Thank you for caring and providing alternative approaches and suggestions for our health and for sharing your expertise with my family. Thank you for Reiki, Body Talk, osteopathy, integrative care, homeopathy, massage, acupuncture, Chinese medicine, craniosacral, tuning forks, singing bowls, and all of the other approaches we tried.

Benny, you never stopped asking or caring about my book, so here it is, Daddy. You have made so much in my life possible. I thank you so much for being there for me and adding the icing on *this* cake—I love you. Love always, teenager.

Jennifer Lopez, you always inspire me. You have been so nurturing and truly supportive and a *real* dear friend to me. You always amaze me with being able to be all you are and do all you do so successfully and so effortlessly. You have always been my idol, my style icon, my E.T., and more. Thank you for sharing yourself with me. Your precious time and commitment to write the foreword for this book mean more to me than any words I can possibly express. I am so grateful and blessed for that, too. Thank you—I Love you, Mama.

Dr. Holly, what a special person you are to me and my family. Thank you for sharing your words in the letter included in this book with me and all the readers in the world. I respect and adore you. Thank you for your time, writing such a meaningful letter, and for being so supportive from the day we met, years ago. I am so appreciative and thankful for you, xo.

Chef Chrisi, you were such a huge force behind me in helping us get on the right bill of health. Thank you for caring for my children's health, and for your interest and passion in health. Many many thank-yous, xo.

Chef Isabell, thank you for nourishing me well through the completion of this passion of mine. I miss those nori veggie wraps. ☺

Jan Miller, first, thank God the dress code for the Legends Ball was black and white; you and I started as a result of a polka-dot dress. You, my friend, are rare. I thank you for being this incredible human being and for sharing the wonderful talents you possess. You are an amazing force of everything. I thank you for *believing* in me, for hanging in there with me for so many years, for understanding this book, understanding me, and seeing my passion and my vision. I thank you for sharing your craft and being great at it. I am truly grateful for you. This is a result of *you* being the best at what you do. I love and adore you. Thank you. Love, Erica.

Dupree, Miller, and Associates—the make-it-happen team. Nena, Nikki, and everyone else, you all helped make this exist, and always kept pushing for this to happen and to have the right home. I thank you all, xo.

Michele Bender, we survived it. Can you believe it? Through the *Annie* rehearsals/play, neurologist appointments, a taxi car accident, acupuncture appointments, knee issues, physical therapy, a trip to the DR, a surprise parents' anniversary party, kids' birthday parties, school pick ups/drop offs, after school activities, spring breaks, *no* fulltime child care, snow days, school projects, Palm Springs, and more. You, Michele, being the mother you are, understood me, heard me, and got it. Thank you for being there through *every* step of the way and for never letting me see or feel your stress. I enjoyed sharing this journey with you so much and I thank you for being there for me and for your dedication. I thank you dearly, Michele; you are amazing and so on point and on top of your game. I learned what I am capable of with the right team player. *Thank you,* xo!

Jonathan, thank you for your help in making the first steps of all of this possible. I am very grateful for your assistance. Thank you.

Ms. Lisa Bonner, thank you for making sure I crossed all *t*'s and dotted all *i*'s. Thank you for your hard work no matter where in the world you were, and for taking this seriously and letting me know it was a priority for you as well. Thank you, Lisa.

Jill, thank you for taking the time to test the recipes and for making sure they were up to par. I appreciate your time and great efforts. Thank you so much.

The book beauty team for my personal photo: Mylah, such a talent at applying makeup. Thank you for pulling this impeccable team together for me at the very last minute. Thank you to the great hair master, Larry; and to Gomillion and Leupold Studios, Steven and Dennis, you *all* are *amazing* and I *love* what you did for me. Your hearts are the reason why you will continue to climb upward, thank you, xo.

To *all* the special individuals at Hachette Book Group and Center Street: What a real blessing to have my first book grace through your hands. I thank you all for all your time, hard work, and hanging in there through challenging moments. Thank you Rolf, Harry, Barbara, Adrienne, Adlai, Jody, Siri, Andrea, Gina, Shannon, Sarah, and more. Thank you from the bottom of my heart for being so hands on with this particular book, for your dedication, your expertise, and for making it a reality for me and all the readers of the world. *The Thriving Child* exists because of all of you and I am grateful to be given this opportunity. This experience was incredible because of the process with the team players, so thank you kindly.

And to all of you who follow me on Twitter and on various other social media, who patiently waited for this book and who continue to support me, I thank you. You all *rock*! Claim what you desire to attain.

To the universe and the stars: Thank you, thank you, thank you for aligning it all in order for me.

Much love and many blessings,

Erica

Index